Dr. Ruth's Guide for the Alzheimer's Caregiver

How to Care for Your Loved One without Getting
Overwhelmed ... and without Doing It All Yourself

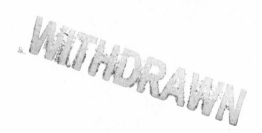

DR. RUTH'S GUIDE FOR THE ALZHEIMER'S CAREGIVER

How to Care for Your Loved One without Getting
Overwhelmed ... and without Doing It All Yourself

Dr. Ruth K. Westheimer

with Pierre A. Lehu

Fresno, California

Published by Quill Driver Books
An imprint of Linden Publishing
2006 South Mary Street, Fresno, California 93721
(559) 233-6633 / (800) 345-4447
QuillDriverBooks.com

cover image © Peter Maszlen—Fotolia.com
cover design: Andrea C. Cooper

Quill Driver Books and Colophon are trademarks of
Linden Publishing, Inc.

ISBN 978-1-61035-135-5

135798642

Printed in the United States of America
on acid-free paper.

Library of Congress Cataloging-in-Publication Data

Westheimer, Ruth K. (Ruth Karola), 1928-
  Dr. Ruth's guide for the Alzheimer's caregiver : how to care for your loved
one without getting overwhelmed and without doing it all by yourself / by
Ruth Westheimer with Pierre Lehu.
     p. cm.
  Includes bibliographical references and index.
  ISBN 978-1-61035-135-5 (pbk. : alk. paper)
  1. Alzheimer's disease--Patients--Care. 2. Alzheimer's disease--Patients-
-Family relationships. I. Lehu, Pierre A. II. Title.
  RC523.W463 2012
  616.8'31--dc23
                          2012030249

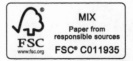

Contents

This book is dedicated to the more than 15 million unpaid caregivers of those with Alzheimer's, who are coping with a great burden, both physically and emotionally.

"The truth of being human is gratitude, the secret of existence is appreciation, its significance is revealed in reciprocity."
—*Insecurity of Freedom*, by Abraham Joshua Heschel, Schocken Press, 1959

Acknowledgments

Dr. Ruth K. Westheimer's acknowledgments:

To the memory of my entire family who perished during the Holocaust. To the memory of my late husband, Fred, who encouraged me in all my endeavors. To my current family, my daughter Miriam Westheimer, Ed.D., son-in-law Joel Einleger, M.B.A., their children Ari and Leora, my son Joel Westheimer, Ph.D., daughter-in-law Barbara Leckie, Ph.D., and their children Michal and Benjamin. I have the best grandchildren in the entire world!

Thanks to all the many family members and friends for adding so much to my life. I'd need an entire chapter to list them all, but some must be mentioned here: Pierre Lehu and I have now collaborated on well over a dozen books, he's the best Minister of Communications I could have asked for! Cliff Rubin, my assistant, thanks! Mark Agronin, M.D., Dr. Peter & Naomi Banks, Peter Berger, M.D., Simon Bergson, Nate Berkus, David Best, M.D., Chuck Blazer, Frank Chervenak, M.D., Richard Cohen, M.D., Martin Englisher, Cynthia Fuchs Epstein, Ph.D., Howard Epstein, Meyer Glaser, David Goslin, Ph.D., Hartmut Grossman, Amos Grunebaum, M.D., Richard & Elaine Heffner, Polly & Herman Hochberg, David Hryck, Esq., Steve Kaplan, Ph.D., Rabbi Barry Dov & Shoshi Katz, Bonnie Kaye, Patti Kenner, Robert Krasner, M.D., Nathan Kravetz, Ph.D., Evelyn Kravetz, Marga & Bill Kunreuther, Dean Stephen Lassonde, Ph.D., Matthew & Vivan Lazar, Rabbi & Mrs. William Lebeau, Robin & Rosemary Leckie, Hope Jensen Leichter, Ph.D., Lou Lieberman, Ph.D., and Mary Cuadrado, Ph.D., Jeff & Nancy Jane Loew, John & Ginger Lollos, Sanford Lopater, Ph.D., & Susan Lopater,

David Marwell, Peter Niculescu, Dale Ordes, Rabbi James & Elana Ponet, Leslie Rahl, Bob & Yvette Rose, Debra Jo Rupp, Larry & Camille Ruvo, Simeon & Rose Schreiber, Daniel Schwartz, Amir Shaviv, David Simon, M.D., Jerry Singerman, Ph.D., Betsy Sledge, William Sledge, M.D., Mark St. Germain, Henry and Sherri Stein, Jeff Tabak, Esq., Marilyn Tabak, Malcolm Thomson, William Turner, M.D., Greg Willenborg, and to all of the people who worked so hard to bring this book into print at Quill Driver Books, especially Steve Mettee, publisher Kent Sorsky, and Jaguar Bennett.

Pierre A. Lehu's acknowledgments:

Thanks to my wife, Joanne Seminara, who not only provided her usual support, but on this book added her legal expertise; my son Peter, daughter-in-law Melissa Sullivan, and fantastic grandson, Jude Sullivan Lehu; my daughter Gabrielle and her future husband, Jim Frawley; my in-laws, Joe and Anita Seminara and the entire Seminara clan. And, of course, a great big thanks to Dr. Ruth. This is our 18th book together and, as she always reminds me, in the Jewish tradition 18 is a lucky number—so good luck to both of us.

Special Thanks to the Wonderful People at the Hebrew SeniorLife Dementia Research, Medical & Care Team Dinner:

Tara Fleming Caruso, MA, LMHC
Jane Givens, M.D., MSCE
Susan Kalish, M.D., MPH
Ruth Kandel, M.D.
Diana Miller, MSW, LICSW
Susan L. Mitchell M.D., MPH
Robert J. Schreiber M.D.
Sheila Trugman, M.D.
Anne M. Thomas
Mary Miller

Special Acknowledgement for having provided materials and for their pioneering effort in research to The Cleveland Clinic Lou Ruvo Center for Brain Health.

Introduction

L ife is always difficult when a loved one is sick, but it's especially so if you are the primary caregiver. And it would be wrong to try to compare the difficulties of caring for someone with one disease to another. If you are under duress, then what you are going through is unique to you and, as far as you are concerned, what other people are going through has no bearing on your life. Yet, it must be acknowledged that the challenges facing caregivers who are dealing with Alzheimer's disease are enormous. If you are responsible for taking care of someone with Alzheimer's, especially in the advanced stages, you have quite a weight on your shoulders. The purpose of this book is to make carrying that weight a bit more tolerable.

Sadly, you are not alone. With almost six million people diagnosed with Alzheimer's disease in the United States, there are an estimated fifteen million caregivers, a number that would equal the fifth-largest state in the nation. The caregivers I'm speaking of are unpaid, meaning the vast majority of them are family members. According to statistics from the *2011 Alzheimer's Disease Facts and Figures*, caregivers provide seventeen billion hours of unpaid care a year, at a cost of over $183 billion. While caregivers bear most of the cost—monetarily, emotionally, and in so many other ways—this is a burden that all of us need to share to some degree, because it can be just too much for the individual caregivers. So to do my part I wrote this book.

It's understandable that your first reaction to seeing this book might be, "Dr. Ruth may be a world renowned expert on sex, but what does she know about taking care of someone with Alzheimer's?" That's a legitimate question and so let me answer it. Thankfully, I have not had to deal with caring for a loved one with Alzheimer's. But a number of friends who do share this burden have come to lean on me for advice. When they told me what they were experiencing, I started asking them questions, just as I do when people come to me with a problem about their sex life or their relationship, and I gave them guidance, which they've told me over and over again that they've found very useful. I'm hopeful that what I learned in the process, together with my training in counseling, will help the caregivers who read this book.

My training is in behavioral therapy. I happened to specialize in the area of sex, but the concept of behavioral therapy is effective in many different aspects of life. A behavioral therapist doesn't concentrate on the underlying cause of a problem, like a psychiatrist or psychologist might do, but offers practical advice on what to do to overcome the problem at hand. And, let's face it: If you are taking care of someone with Alzheimer's, you have your share of problems. So what I am going to do in this book is offer practical advice on how to cope with your particular burden. I'm going to show you how to get help, even if you are reluctant about asking for it. I'm going to offer you advice on how to work with your family, despite any fraying of relationships Alzheimer's may have caused.

Much of the specific technical information about Alzheimer's disease in this book can be found elsewhere. I have every intention of standing on the shoulders of those who have a lot more experience dealing with Alzheimer's patients than I do. In fact, the second half of this book relies mostly on information I've gleaned from other sources. Some of this material comes from actual friends and acquaintances of mine. (I have a friend who uses me to raise money for Alzheimer's research, and some very generous friends of his have bid as much as $100,000 to have lunch with me to show their support for this cause.) Much of the advice I offer here comes from the research I've done, which you could do on your own. But the problem with doing your own research is that you are likely to become overwhelmed with information at a time when you are already overwhelmed with the duties of being a caregiver.

So what I hope to do with this book is to concisely present the information that will help you to cope. My advice is influenced by all that I've learned about human behavior, both while training and during my thirty-plus years as a therapist. It is advice that I feel will be fully beneficial and useful to you.

When a couple comes to me with a sexual problem, I give them "homework." The reason they listen to me and do what I say is because they've seen me in action over the years and trust me to steer them in the right direction. I have been very careful over the last thirty years to never sensationalize my area of expertise, to never lower my principles one inch to profit from or abuse the field of sex therapy. That's why people respect me. No one has ever heard me say one word about the myriad sex scandals that crop up year after year, because as I see it, these are none of my business. I'm not the least bit interested in getting media attention, as much as I might love it, on the back of someone else. I also have never treated real people on television, which I believe will only worsen their problem. On my TV shows, I had actors portray someone with a problem. So, you see, I have set very high standards for myself and I don't ever lower them.

Thus, when it comes to digesting all the information out there on Alzheimer's for your benefit, you can be sure I'm not going to offer you the latest or the most sensational advice unless I am one 100 percent sure that it is beneficial.

I have a doctorate in education. I am not a medical doctor and I never hesitate to remind people of this. In my books and newspaper column, I say it again and again; I don't offer medical opinions. I do consult experts and I will quote them, but let me say you're not going to be reading very much in this book about the latest treatments for Alzheimer's. I don't have the knowledge or expertise to assess these, and whenever I don't know something, I keep my mouth tightly shut. But if I do tell you to try something, you can be sure that in my heart and soul I believe that it can potentially help you. Again, I want to emphasize that I'm writing this book for you, the caregiver, not for the patient. I want to offer you advice, solace, inspiration, strength, and courage so that you can continue your duties as caretaker and still maintain the highest quality of life for yourself as possible.

At the age of ten, my mother and grandmother put me on a train to Switzerland to escape the Holocaust, along with three hundred other German Jewish children. Though I didn't know it at the time, I would never see my family again. I cried while on that train, a lot, but then I led the other children in song to help lift their spirits. I give you this story to show that it's not an accident that I became Dr. Ruth. Somewhere inside me a fire burns to help people overcome their problems. And though I'm eighty-four now, that fire burns just as strongly, and through this book I hope that I can offer you some of the warmth of that fire to help you make the best of this most difficult situation you now find yourself in.

PART ONE:

ADVICE FROM DR. RUTH

1

How to Help Yourself

It's not easy taking care of a patient with Alzheimer's disease, particularly if the patient is living at home, in which case caretaking is, for all intents and purposes, a full-time job. You can't ever really let your guard down because the unexpected soon becomes the expected. Patterns that your loved one seems to follow may change overnight. And if the person you're caring for is a sundowner (a patient who's confusion intensifies as the sun sets and evening approaches), then your nights may be worse than your days. At the same time, all this is happening not to some stranger that you're paid to take care of, but to someone, if it's a parent, with whom you've spent your entire life, and, no matter what the relationship, someone whom you love dearly.

One of the people whom I've been advising has a wife with Alzheimer's. He reports that the worst aspect for him is that he has nobody to talk to about what's happening. For some fifty years they always shared everything, the good and the bad, but now when he most needs to talk to his wife about what he's going through, she's not available to him, even though she's in the same room as he is.

It's true that having an emotional attachment with the patient is helpful to you. Let's face it: In all probability, no amount of money in the world would get you to take on the duties of a caregiver for an Alzheimer's patient 24/7. So the fact that it's your mother, your father, your spouse, or a sibling gives you strength that you otherwise wouldn't have. But that love may also push you beyond your limits.

Given all that caregivers go through, not surprisingly studies have shown that caregivers suffer both emotionally and physically. More than

60 percent of caregivers report high levels of stress. And because someone with Alzheimer's can live a very long time, relief from this stress may seem impossible to attain, multiplying its impact. (In fact, according to the *Journal of the American Medical Association*, a majority of caregivers predecease the person for whom they are caring, which in part is due to that stress.) In addition, sleep deprivation, when present, adds to the deleterious effects of all that stress.

But stress isn't the only issue. Thirty percent of caregivers report feeling depressed. Stress combined with depression often leads to other health problems. The cost of treating these caregivers for the problems caused by the increased stress in their lives is estimated to be eight billion dollars annually. Thus, relieving yourself of any portion of this stress is vital not only to your emotional well-being but to your very health. So, let's delve into ways of reducing stress in your life.

Avoid Drawing Lines in the Sand

Let's say you have a favorite TV program. Let's pretend it's *NCIS*, and at some time during the day, maybe when you're particularly tired or exasperated, you say to yourself, "Tonight I'm watching *NCIS* come hell or high water because I deserve a break." This type of reaction makes perfect sense. Offering yourself a carrot at the end of a long day, knowing that you're going to get a reward for all your hard work, might make it easier to get through the day. And in many situations, I would tell you to do just that. But not in your situation, and I will explain why this is the case.

This type of goal is like drawing a line in the sand. You're saying to yourself, "I'm going to fight as hard as I can to make sure that my life as the caregiver of an Alzheimer's patient is not going to stop me from watching my favorite TV show tonight." But what happens if, at 8:00 P.M. that night when *NCIS* is supposed to air, your spouse has a crisis of some sort? Are you going to lock him or her in a padded room and say, "Tough luck, I'm watching my show?" What's going to happen is that you're going to do whatever it is that your spouse requires to be done, but while you're doing it, you're going to be very upset because after spending all day waiting to watch *NCIS*, you're going to miss out on this reward. At 8:00 P.M., you'll be doing what you already did ten times that day, but because it's causing you to cross that line in the sand that you drew, it's going to make you feel very frustrated.

So, here's my first rule when it comes to taking care of someone with Alzheimer's: Don't draw lines in the sand. It doesn't matter whether or not you tell an Alzheimer's patient you want to watch *NCIS* that night, because, for many, their short-term memory is so deteriorated that even if you told them a dozen times they wouldn't remember it.

While nobody can say this occurs for sure, I know that many caregivers will swear that an Alzheimer's patient seems to know exactly what to do to push your buttons. Such patients seem to have a sixth sense about doing things that drive you crazy. They probably don't, but who knows, maybe they do. Maybe they sense when you're not paying full attention to them and somehow that sets them off and they act up.

People with Alzheimer's lose most or all of their sense of inhibition, so where a normal person might not be so demanding all the time, understanding that a caregiver needs a break, someone with Alzheimer's doesn't have that particular filter. If they want something, they demand it, just like an infant. Whatever the cause, the reality—part of your reality—is that rather than drawing lines in the sand, you have to figure out how to get around such situations. Similar to how many forms of martial arts teach you how to defend against a particular line of attack, or like in the game of chess, where there is a particular way of defending against an attack by your opponent, by being prepared, you can offset the damage, and if you are able to do that day after day, you'll find that caring for your loved one is less stress-inducing.

The simple way of protecting yourself against the particular problem I just posed is to make sure that you record that favorite program of yours so that if you can't watch it when it's actually airing, you can watch it when you do have some time to spare later on. By being proactive, you can save yourself a large dose of stress.

Other ways of being proactive might include never allowing yourself to run out of basic food supplies, like coffee for your morning fix. You might want to set your watch ahead by ten, fifteen, or even thirty minutes so that when you have an appointment, you'll be less likely to encounter the stress that comes from being late. Deadlines, you see, whether for a favorite show, a store that's going to close, or a doctor's appointment are your enemy. They're likely to cause you added stress. So keep a careful watch on the horizon for looming deadlines and then do whatever you can to lessen the impact on your emotions if it turns out that you have missed one.

One particularly powerful way of defusing a potentially stressful situation caused by a deadline is to make sure that you're getting as much help as possible.

Accept Every Offer of Help

I'm sure that you have friends, neighbors, or relatives who say to you, "Please tell me how I can be of help." Now, many of these people lead busy lives, and while their intentions are good, there really is not that much they can do for you on a day-to-day basis. But they honestly do want to help you—in fact, it would make them feel good if they could help you—so rather than saying, "Thanks but I can handle it," give them little chores that, when added up, will make your day a little easier for you.

So let's go back to our *NCIS* example. I've told you that you should record the show so that you can watch it later. But maybe you're not that technically savvy. Or, having to remember every little detail of how to operate the technology becomes too burdensome, and so you end up not doing it and then mope because you missed your show. Here's a simple chore that you could pass off to someone else. If you tell one of these people who say they want to help that there are some shows that you don't want to miss and would they mind recording them, I'm sure that they'll jump at the chance. They want to help, and this task is a really easy one, not adding much of a burden to their life at all. You'll feel better knowing that you have "*NCIS* insurance," which will make your day a little easier. And even if you end up being able to watch the show when it airs, when your friend or neighbor presents you with the recording, just knowing that they were thinking of you, that you're not all alone in dotting every I and crossing every T, will brighten your day a little.

Now I've used one little example of a chore you could pass on, but there are many, many more.

Consider shopping: I'm sure you have a neighbor or friend who would feel good knowing that each time he went to the supermarket, he was helping you out by getting some items for you. When he makes his delivery, you'll get to see him, even only briefly, which will make you feel good and brighten your day.

Consider cooking: Let's say you have a neighbor, and once a week she makes roast beef for dinner. It wouldn't add much work for her to make a roast that was a few pounds larger and give the extra portion to you. Of course you'd pay her for the difference in price, but at least that would be one meal you wouldn't have to worry about. Get three neighbors involved (some extra tuna casserole or mac and cheese on Tuesdays, fish on Fridays, etc.) and you'll have quite a burden lifted from your shoulders for very little effort on the part of those who have volunteered to help out.

Consider hair appointments: When it's time for you to get your hair cut, dyed, or whatever, choose a friend or neighbor with whom you'll coordinate your appointment and who will stay at your home during that time.

Consider hobbies: If you have a hobby and need some time off to enjoy it, designate one friend whose job it is to fill in for you when you take some time for yourself. Hobbies can be a very important channel for relieving stress. Spend a couple of hours fishing or gardening or playing bridge and it will be much easier to return to your duties as caregiver. A rewarding hobby isn't frivolous—it can be a potent tonic that will give you renewed energy.

Consider a last minute fill-in: There are going to be times when you will be running late. You said you'd be home at five, but … a zillion things could come up. A designated pinch hitter for those times will be a life-saver.

Now at first glance you may be saying, "Dr. Ruth, come on, I can't go asking people to volunteer for such small, focused tasks. It seems silly." It may seem silly, but it's not silly at all. Instead it's very practical for several reasons.

The first is that you may have some people who you really rely on to help you regularly, like a close relative, a sister or brother, son or daughter. And they're great and give you a lot of their free time, and that's wonderful. While it may appear to be a burden on them, you want to be able to call them guilt-free when you really need them. By reassigning some little chores that they might otherwise be doing, such as coming over when you need to get your hair taken care of, you're sending them a very practical message that you do appreciate how much they're helping, and you're trying to do what you can to make it easier on them.

This also gives you a measure of independence. Engaging a number of people to provide assistance in small ways can help you feel less dependent overall. Every chance you get to find help in other ways will make you feel more independent, and thus help you to feel better about yourself.

Finally, there is no truer axiom than "Giving is receiving." It really does make people feel better to give of themselves. Obviously, with everyone so busy these days, it's impossible for most of the people who offer to help you to give very much of themselves. But to give you an hour on Saturday morning every couple of weeks so that you can tend to a personal need like getting your hair done might be the perfect way for allowing people to get that feeling of satisfaction that comes from doing good. And maybe you can find two or three people to share this duty, so that it really isn't much of a burden for any one of them.

My overall point here is not to always say, "No, but thank you" when someone offers to help you out, but to see if you can utilize a little bit of their time in some simple way. I assure you it will be a win-win for everyone—for you, for those who help you out most often, and for the person who can give a little bit of their time to make your life slightly easier.

A Help Registry

Having read many blogs and other reports from caregivers, I know that one complaint caregivers have is that most offers of help fall by the wayside. Is this because those offering are only saying what they think they should be saying? Sometimes that may be true, but I also think it's because there's not enough follow-through. The person offering to help doesn't know exactly what is needed, and the caregiver may be too embarrassed to ask for something specific, even something as simple as the suggestions I've been making. So here's some advice on how to get around this conundrum, so that when someone offers you help you can make use of them.

When a couple gets married these days, they usually register with retail or online establishments that have a bridal registry. Those who want to give them a gift can go to the store, call, or, most likely, go online and buy a gift for the couple that they've actually requested, so that the couple doesn't end up with a shopping cart full of useless or duplicate gifts that the newlyweds have to return when they get back from their honeymoon. I think this concept can be used by caregivers.

Make a list of all the things you could use help with. Make sure that you've chosen tasks that will take very little time, and maybe only need doing once, as well as tasks that take longer and would be repeated, like the tasks I've listed above. You can do several things with this list. If you are computer literate, or if you have a relative or friend who is, you can post the list on the Web on a blog, where people can sign up for various tasks. You could also hand out this list to anyone who offers their assistance, or you can ask for their address and mail it to them later. And, if you're too embarrassed to ask for help, get someone else to take charge of bringing volunteers into your life (that would then be their contribution). Obviously, nobody would be forced into signing up to take on one of the tasks, but you certainly would get more actual help with such a list of specific needs than without it. Once you have a sign-up list in place, when someone offered you help, you'll have a simple method of turning such offers into actual help.

By the way, with such a registry, you might be able to recruit people you don't know very well or those who have never expressed an offer of help but would actually like to contribute. For example, houses of worship could keep such lists on a bulletin board near the door so that, after service, members of the congregation could review them and see if there were a job that they would be willing to take on. Such lists could also be posted at places of employment, either where you work or have worked previously, or where family members work. Your registry could also be given to other groups, like the Boy Scouts and Girl Scouts, and organizations like the Lions Club or Kiwanis. I understand that you wouldn't want total strangers coming into your home without some way of vetting them, but I think that if such a registry is posted through the types of organizations I've listed above, you wouldn't have to be overly concerned with the caliber of people you would attract.

Of course, if a total stranger comes to help you in some way, you're going to want to be a little careful. Make sure that you get some information about them before they enter the picture. Find out how they learned of the registry. If they go to the same house of worship you go to, for example, you can easily ask someone there about them. But if they don't have any connection whatsoever that you can check, then you need to be extra cautious. In any case, if you're having people you don't know very well coming into your house, and that includes hired help, I'd make sure to place any valuable jewelry in a safe deposit box and store your silver at the home of a relative.

Reciprocity

Even though you clearly are deserving of help, as someone who's always been independent it's understandable that you might feel a little awkward about getting other people to lend you a hand. Accepting charity is an admission that you need assistance, and that is a hard thing for anyone to ask for. Independence is something we all treasure and giving any of your independence up can be unsettling. What you have to do is put yourself in the shoes of the person offering this assistance. Imagine yourself doing something similar. What emotions would you be feeling? Would you think the person you were helping was weak, or would you recognize how strong they were for accepting this role of caregiver? Would you be helping them out of a sense of pity or admiration? I'm sure in either case it would be the latter, and you have to realize that anyone who helps you will be feeling the same way about you.

Of course, it might help you to feel better about having to accept someone's help if you could reciprocate in some way. Obviously, your time is limited, but that doesn't mean that you couldn't find a way to repay these volunteers in small ways. You could bake cookies, do some sewing for them if you're good at that type of thing, make phone calls to one of their favorite charities, put a sign in your lawn for a candidate they support, baby-sit, or accept packages for people who work during the day. In order to reciprocate, you must think creatively.

If you have a skill that people can really use, like the ability to knit a sweater or prepare a tax return or tutor a language, you may be able to share your expertise in return for assistance via time-banking organizations. There are many cities around the country that have groups taking part in this concept, and you can easily see if there is one near you and learn more about the concept by going to www.timebanks.org. (If you are not computer literate, ask someone you know to print out the information.)

And let's not forget that by having people help you, and helping them in return, you'll increase your level of contact with the outside world. A common complaint among caregivers is that they spend so many hours with a care recipient who can't interact in normal ways, which can be isolating and lonely for the caregiver.

Let's consider some specific ways people could help you.

Consider going to the library: Find someone who understands your taste in books and trust them to pick one out for you every two weeks. Or, if you prefer to buy books, they could shop for you. If you don't have a computer, someone could order books for you via Amazon or Barnes & Noble to be delivered right to your door.

Consider picking up prescriptions: Let the pharmacist know that your helpmate person is authorized to sign for you.

Consider accepting packages: Ordering items online may be the easiest way for you to shop, but you can never tell when a delivery man will arrive. If you're giving your spouse a bath, for example, not having to answer the doorbell would be a blessing. So, if you could use a neighbor's address for your packages, that could prove useful.

Consider activities with your spouse: If your spouse is calm when being read to, having one or more people come in to read to your spouse for half an hour will free up your time to do something else. Many people with Alzheimer's like to look at old pictures. A volunteer who reads to your care recipient might also review family photo albums with them.

Volunteers with artistic talent or interests could also be very useful. Often the parts of the brain that are used to appreciate art, which includes looking at images and listening to music, are not as badly damaged as other areas. So someone who could come to your house and play a musical instrument or help your care recipient paint or sing might make a very important contribution. He or she would likely feel very good about putting such talents to work in order to help someone with Alzheimer's.

Consider filling your gas tank: Since you never know when you might have to drive somewhere, to a hospital, let's say, you never want your tank to be even close to empty. This is a chore that takes only a few minutes, so it would certainly not place much of a burden on anyone interested in helping you.

I must mention here that you should have a ready supply of cash in the house so that you can repay your friends for such expenses, unless there are particular cases when you can just give them your credit card.

Consider sending your mail: If you live in an apartment where you can't simply put the mail in your box for the postman, this small chore could be important.

Consider depositing checks: This is a simple chore for a friend to do for you.

Consider going to the cleaners: This is another simple chore that a friend might eagerly assist with.

I'm not suggesting that this list of helping-hand activities is exhaustive. I just want to give you some examples so that you can examine your own day-to-day activities and using a little creativity to discover times during the day when help would make life a little easier for you. Of course, you might even need help in coming up with this list. You know the saying: "You can't see the forest for the trees." You might not be able to see how an outsider could help you to do some of the things you do, but maybe someone else could do so. If you're having a hard time figuring out where you could use assistance or can only come up with excuses as to why you really don't need any help, ask a close relative or friend to sit down with you and examine the question of how volunteers might be able to be of use to you.

Chores Are Chores

I understand that you will often be looking for opportunities to get out of the house, and I encourage you to do that. But don't look at doing chores as your only means of escape. Don't hold on to doing chores just because you think that if you don't have a "legitimate" excuse to leave the house, like going shopping or to the cleaners, you'll feel too guilty to go out at all. That's not a helpful attitude. You deserve breaks, and those breaks can be frivolous; they shouldn't have to involve chores. If others are willing to relieve you of some chores, accept this help gladly. Remember they're going to feel good about helping you. And, when you have time to take a walk on a sunny day, don't feel guilty because you're not "doing" anything. No one will resent you for this. People who see you will think, "Good for you," and they will recognize that there but for fate, it could be them.

Remember that if anyone who is helping you seems to resent that you are "just" going out for a breath of fresh air (or to the movies or ice-skating), that person has a problem, not you.

Of course, there are people who will offer you help but will then let you down. That's one reason to dole out small chores, so that if anyone who volunteers ends up being unreliable, you won't be left stranded having to do something important. (This is one reason I didn't mention such duties as driving the care recipient to the doctor. If this is something you can't do yourself, it should be delegated only to either someone close to you, whom you trust completely, or to a professional service, such as a taxi or ambulette.)

This chapter assumes that people are offering to help you, but that might not be the case. Don't worry about that now; I'll be talking more about how to get help in another chapter. If you are getting lots of offers of help, you can skip the parts about getting help when you reach them later in the book.

So, it's time to recap what's been covered in this chapter. The first thing is that I want you to remain as flexible as possible and not to draw any lines in the sand. This will spare you endless frustration.

The second thing is that there are people who honestly want to help you because they've learned the important lesson in life that doing good offers unrivaled rewards in terms of satisfaction. Accept such offers, but devise a good system, such as a sign-up list, to help these good souls help you. Make a list of tasks that are simple and won't take up a lot of anyone's time, so that when you get an offer of help, you're ready to accept it.

Finally, understand that you will be disappointed from time to time. If you're at your very limits in terms of physical and psychological energy, such disappointments can be very hard on you. It's OK to feel sad and upset for a short time if someone disappoints you, but then I want you to put any such bad experiences aside and concentrate on all the good in your life.

2

Feelings

I ended the previous chapter by talking about disappointment, but, of course, there are a whole range of human emotions, and if you're caring for a loved one with a serious illness, you're going to go through all of them.

Feelings are unavoidable. That may sound obvious, but you'd be surprised at how many people try to suppress their feelings, mostly bad ones, but even at times some good ones. There are people who, when given a present, don't feel good but feel bad. They think they don't deserve the gift. So, rather than smiling and saying thank you, they'll show almost no expression at all, in part because they don't understand their own feelings well enough to articulate them. But even people who don't appear to show any feelings still experience feelings. As I said, feelings are unavoidable.

However, feelings, though unavoidable, can be repressed. In those cases, as soon as you begin to feel sad, angry, guilty, happy, aroused, in love, hateful, envious, jealous, and so on, you can teach yourself to stuff those feelings back where they came from. For many people, repressing feelings seems to be the best possible coping mechanism for a distressing situation. If you have just lost someone you love, in our society you won't feel comfortable walking around the mall with tears streaming down your face. Perhaps, however, it would be better, healthier, if you did just that, but peer pressure exerts a very strong influence on all of us. In your current situation, in dealing with someone with Alzheimer's, you've got enough on your plate without trying to cast off the social rules by which we live. The trick that you must learn is to maintain appearances but not repress your feelings entirely.

Strong emotions that never get expressed are extremely damaging. If you've lost someone you love, you must mourn. You must spend some time crying and sobbing and fully experiencing the sadness that comes from losing a loved one. Why is this so important? It's because you can't repress some feelings without inadvertently repressing others. If you are successful at keeping yourself from being sad, by the same token, you will not experience being happy. You see, what people who repress their feelings soon learn is that when you open yourself up to one feeling—let's say happiness—then other feelings, like sadness, are likely to escape as well. So, if you are trying to keep yourself from experiencing sadness, you will likely end up becoming numb to other emotions.

Then there are people who attempt to numb themselves by turning to alcohol or drugs. This is a much bigger problem and not really within the scope of this book, but I must point this out. If you are turning to alcohol or drugs in order to cope with your caregiving duties, you need to get professional help. I'm not talking about having a drink when you come home in order to make you a bit more relaxed. That's perfectly fine (assuming you're not an alcoholic). I'm talking about using a substance to make yourself emotionally numb for long periods of time.

You have to find a happy medium for your feelings. That's a bit of a strange phrase for this discussion—"happy medium"—but then again it isn't, because in the end what I want is for you to be able to experience the greatest degree of happiness that you can.

GUILT

When a loved one is ill, most of us may feel guilty, even if we have absolutely no reason to feel guilty. I read a story in the *New York Times* about a man whose father began to suffer from Alzheimer's. Because the man was afraid that he would get it too, he took something like seventy-five different vitamins and supplements a day. He exercised. He did all sorts of word puzzles. In short, he took every precaution possible, and yet, in the end, he fell victim to Alzheimer's.

What this story illustrates is that Alzheimer's is not something that you, as the husband or wife, son or daughter, or sister or brother of one of its victims has any power to prevent. If you happened to have an elderly parent who took a fall in the bathtub, and you'd been meaning to install some extra bars for them to hold onto, there would be a legitimate reason to feel guilty. My co-author Pierre's mother felt incredibly guilty that she wasn't by her husband's side when he passed away during his first night in a hospice. She'd been told he would live for a couple of weeks, so she'd gone home to bed that night. In cases like these, there is some realistic rationale for feeling guilty, and that guilt can be very hard to overcome. But with Alzheimer's guilt has no place, because there is nothing—zero— that you could have done to prevent it. Yet, you are always likely to feel guilty, guilty that your loved one came down with this terrible disease and guilty each time he or she reaches a new stage of deterioration.

One reaction to this guilt is to totally repress it. When the feeling of guilt comes over you, you just stuff it back down. From a purely practical point of view, that makes sense. There is no reason to feel guilty, so why should you allow yourself to feel guilty? But here's a good reason: If you stuff those guilty feelings back inside, you won't be dealing with them. They'll keep coming back, and since we've seen that you can't stuff down just one emotion, stuffing these feelings of guilt will cause you to stuff down emotions that are appropriate. So what should you do? You should allow yourself to feel guilty. But guilty about what? You couldn't have done anything to stop the progression of Alzheimer's. That's just the point. If you let the guilty feelings well up temporarily, but they have nothing to hang onto, they'll quickly go away. They'll dissipate and won't bother you. And, while this process will happen more than once, eventually it will stop. In time, you'll stop experiencing these waves of guilt because your brain will come to realize that this guilt is not appropriate.

Often when some people feel this guilt they make a huge mistake. They think that if they're feeling guilty, there must be a good reason for it. Even if they don't know what they might have done wrong—and how could they because they didn't do anything wrong—they will look for a reason to justify the guilty feelings. They'll say to themselves, "Oh, if only I had done this or that." Then instead of dissipating, those guilty feelings will grow stronger and make them more miserable. So it is vital for you to be able to assess whether any feelings of guilt you may be feeling are valid or not. What you should never do is justify guilty feelings that have no validity.

Now you might ask, what is the purpose of guilt? Of course, the main purpose of appropriate guilt is to keep you from doing things that you shouldn't be doing. But what about inappropriate guilt, which occurs when you haven't done anything wrong? In my opinion, such guilt leads to compassion. If a baby is crying, guilt acts as the trigger, the catalyst, to release the feelings of compassion you need to go take care of it. If you didn't feel guilty and hence compassionate, you could just feel angry. You might take it out on that crying baby, or on that dazed Alzheimer's patient. So a little guilt isn't necessarily a bad thing as long as you don't overreact to it, as long as you don't find reasons to feel more guilty and allow this emotion to become all-consuming.

Thus, when it comes to your feelings of guilt, what you must do is assess the situation. If you determine that you have no reason to feel guilty, then accept the feeling, which as I said will become weaker and weaker, and just go about your business of being caretaker to someone who needs you. What may help you to overcome guilty feelings is to write them down. Try to explain to yourself why you're feeling guilty. This can be difficult because there are often no obviously rational reasons, so this exercise will help demonstrate that your feelings of guilt are inappropriate.

Eventually, there may come a particular time when you are going to feel very guilty, and that's if you need to take your loved one to live in a specialized facility. If you hadn't been capable of feeling some realistic degree of guilt, you might have made that decision a lot sooner. It's so incredibly difficult and frustrating taking care of someone with Alzheimer's. Having that burden lifted is something I'm sure you wish for every day. (And, since one way for the burden to be lifted is for the patient to pass away, such a wish is certainly going to trigger a high degree of guilt, but more about that in a second.) So, the following is my advice for dealing with making the decision to send your loved one to a facility of some sort.

The first thing I recommend is to prepare for that day, even if it ends up never coming. Visit some facilities. Ask other people you know who have taken someone to a facility about what the particular facility was like. Do as much research on the Internet as you can. Why am I telling you to do this early on? Because at an early stage, you won't feel guilty. Since it's not something you're planning on doing in the near future, your outlook will be more scientific and rational rather than emotional. If you're at your wits' end, if you're nervous and sleep deprived and wracked with guilt, how easy is it going to be to make the right decisions? But if you have a plan already in place, when the time comes to make this difficult decision the only thing you'll only have to concern yourself with is its timing.

And, of course, there may well be financial considerations. The sooner you plan for these factors, the easier it will be to deal with them at the right time. (The legal and financial aspects of this process are very complicated, and I would strongly urge you to consult with someone with expertise in this area as soon as possible, at the very first diagnosis by a doctor. See Chapter 12 for more information.)

You will likely consult with other family members about the decision to place a loved one in a facility. If you are speaking with them when such a move is imminent, all sorts of emotions may arise to complicate matters. But if you do it early enough (and, again, at this stage you're just discussing which facility would be best), then these discussions will not be quite as emotionally charged.

Of course, there are some people who take a very hard and rational approach to caregiving and don't allow guilt to play much of a role and send their loved one to a facility at a very early stage of the disease. They could have many rationales, from needing to work and not wanting to have to worry about having strangers in their home all day long, to simply deciding that they place more importance on the quality of their own life than that of the person with Alzheimer's, whose quality of life is only going to get worse in any case.

I don't have a problem with that attitude. I don't think that you should make the decision to dedicate years of your life to being a full-time caregiver based on guilt. It should be a rational decision, and if you come to the conclusion that, after weighing all the pluses and minuses, you'd rather not take on such duties, you have my blessings.

I imagine that most people reading this book have decided to be full-time caregivers, and part of their decision may have been based on guilt. That's okay. But if a time comes when you feel that, having experienced caregiving to a certain point, you no longer want to continue such duties, then by all means don't continue this role only because you feel guilty—go ahead and make whatever decision you deem is right for you.

Anger

I'm an impatient person. And when someone is impatient and things aren't going fast enough, his or her reaction is often frustration, which materializes as anger. But I'm also someone who doesn't remember when people have done something to make me angry. I've lived through such horrors that I naturally shunt aside bad memories, so that while I may be very angry at someone at one moment, I'll completely forget about it later. I'm not excusing myself or anyone from becoming angry. It's not the best emotion, but to tell someone not to be angry is useless, because anger is a very strong emotion, and at the particular moment it arises—it's very difficult to keep it tamped down. But when anger is very destructive, it will linger and fester.

Staying angry at someone does you more damage than it does to the other person. Anger causes physical changes in your body, like elevated blood pressure, which, if repeated over and over again, are going to damage you in the long run. So how do you set anger aside? The answer is by actually forcing yourself to put that anger aside. When you start to get angry, you must have some positive thoughts ready to take the place of that anger. Let me give you a concrete example.

Let's say it's your mother who has Alzheimer's. And, let's say as a result of this disease, each time she sees you she says you're fat. Your natural reaction is going to be to become angry at her, as no one likes to be insulted. But you also know that this isn't your mother speaking but her diseased mind. Now, let's say when you were young you went to Disneyland as a family and had a really great time. What I advise you to do each time your mother insults you by saying you're fat is to pull up some of those images of that trip to Disneyland so that you can quickly replace the anger welling up in you with some positive feelings. If you keep doing that, after a time you'll see that you won't get angry when your mother calls you fat. You will have trained your brain not to react negatively to that insult. It may take a week, it may take a month, but if you are determined to overcome this anger, you can do it.

You are also likely to become angry at your loved one for the situation he or she has put the two of you in. While you're unlikely to express that anger, because consciously you know that it's not his or her fault, that doesn't mean you won't feel angry subconsciously, in which case you'll end up expressing that anger in other ways or aiming it at the wrong people. If the clerk at the supermarket is slow, you'll feel angry at him, maybe even lashing out at him verbally, though the real cause of that anger is the condition of your life at the moment.

It's vital that you recognize the real source of such anger so that you don't give in to it. You don't want your personality to change—you don't want to go around being an angry person all the time. Since being angry causes your body to release adrenaline, one way of dissipating this anger is by doing something physical, like going for a walk to burn off steam.

Obviously, the examples I've given you are just that, examples. You're going to have to pay close attention to the various aspects of being a caregiver that make you angry, and then you're to have to carefully assess which type of stimuli will dissipate that anger. It will take some self-discipline. But in the long run, you will be a lot better off. If you really can't cope, then go to a counselor to learn anger management.

HAPPINESS

Being happy is certainly a state that is to be desired, but sometimes it's difficult to be happy because you won't allow yourself to feel good. You may feel guilty about being happy when you have a loved one nearby who is afflicted with Alzheimer's. Or you may steel yourself against feeling sad by building a shell around yourself, which may keep you from feeling sadness but which also prevents you from feeling joy.

If you've had to take on the duties of caregiver, there is no doubt that you bear a great burden, but that doesn't mean that your life has to be devoid of happiness or laughter. As I said earlier, it's better to allow yourself to feel sad once in a while, because that way you can also experience and enjoy happiness when pleasant things occur.

Your happy moments may appear spontaneously, but they may also take some planning. Because your life revolves around that of another, you may need to make actual appointments to harvest some happiness. Let me give you an example. Let's say that you have a friend from childhood who lives out of town, and every time the two of you have a gabfest on the phone, you feel uplifted after hanging up. If you leave it to chance, weeks or even months might go by without the two of you having a chance to really talk. So while it may seem strange to have to schedule time with this person, I'm telling you to do just that. This way, you'll be able to ask someone else to look after the person you are caring for at the time you make the date for the phone chat so that you and your friend will have enough free time to really talk. And by scheduling your phone chat ahead of time, your friend will also have the free time to offer you. Not only will the scheduled conversation make you feel better, but knowing that it is on the horizon will also help you to lift your spirits.

At this point I must also offer a cautionary note. There are some things that you might think make you happy but really don't because they're just not good for you. Some people turn to food when they need comfort. I'm not saying that you should never have an occasional treat, but being a caregiver is a long-haul procedure. If you're going to "reward" yourself with half a pint of ice cream every night, the results such rewards will have on your appearance are not going to make you happy in the long run, nor will ice cream treats do much for your overall health. Some people turn to alcohol, but alcohol is a depressant, so that's certainly not the right direction, not that I have anything against a limited amount of alcohol consumption. Then there's this strange concept of "vegging out" in front of the TV. Ask yourself, have you ever done that and really felt happy afterward? Now I'm not saying you shouldn't watch TV, but do it in a planned manner; don't waste precious minutes and hours of your limited free time. (Of course if your loved one likes watching TV and it keeps them calm, then watching TV may be an activity that allows you to catch your breath while still keeping an eye on him or her. While that's a legitimate use of TV, according to my standards, I'd tell you to use earplugs while you're sitting there and read a good book or write a letter to a friend. But, of course, that's me.)

You know, if there's one lesson that you should take away from caring for someone with dementia, it's that we just don't know how many days are left to us. I've come close to death several times, and perhaps that makes me value life more than most. You'll find me out having dinner, seeing a show, or attending a party just about every night of the week because I abhor the concept of "wasting time." Make the most of each day. When you have free time, use it to squeeze out the most pleasure that you can, not by doing your best imitation of a vegetable.

THE LIGHTER SIDE

As with every aspect of life, there will be moments provided by someone with Alzheimer's that should elicit a smile or two. I heard of one woman who loved the color pink. She was going to move into her daughter's house, and her daughter, busy packing up her mother's belongings, lost track of her for a while. The woman knew that she needed to have her hair dyed, spotted her daughter's pink lipstick, and when the daughter next saw her, she had a head of pink hair that she'd applied herself. Then there was the son whose mother no longer recognized him, and when he'd visit her at the nursing home, she'd say, "Oh, what a handsome young man," and start flirting with him. What else can you do but laugh in such situations?

Of course laughter is not only good for you, but also good for your care recipient. So work at trying to bring as much laughter into your home as possible. Rent comedies and watch them together. Read funny books to your mom. If you know someone who's a fountain of jokes, make sure to ask that person for a daily or weekly supply. You know how babies like to play peek-a-boo? Find actions that will surprise your care recipient and put a smile on his face. Only you know what will work, and if you need to, experiment a bit to see what tickles her funny bone.

Feeling Tired

Your body has a physical need for rest, and so there comes a time every day when you need to go to sleep. But there are people who wake up after eight hours sleep and say that they feel tired. Or else they say it at other times during the day. This is not usually the physical need for rest but rather a psychological phenomenon, and it's one that I don't permit in my life and I don't think you should either. As I just pointed out, we have a very limited time on this earth, and we have no idea when something may happen to either end that time entirely or afflict us in some way that will make the things we love today impossible to recognize or to enjoy tomorrow. So, to my way of thinking, wasting time is a huge mistake. And if you are "feeling" tired rather than being physically tired, most likely you are going to waste time.

I say that when you're "feeling" tired what is actually happening is that you're bored. If you were doing something exciting, that "feeling" of tiredness would disappear in a second. So, when you're "feeling" tired, instead of vegging out in front of the TV or moping about, I want you to do something that will alleviate your boredom. Read a good book or newspaper or magazine. Write a letter or send an e-mail to a friend. If you don't have a hobby, find one and use your spare time to engage in your hobby. Make notes of things you want to know more about and look them up on the Internet. Consider taking a class online. Universities like MIT and many others make their classes available through their websites so that you can take courses taught by world-famous professors without leaving your house. Buy a sketchbook and some pencils and teach your-self to sketch. Learn a new language or a new style of cooking. I could go on and on, but my point is to encourage you to discover things to do that will wake up your mind so that you can banish those tired feelings caused by mental fatigue more than anything else.

If you are the spouse of the person suffering from Alzheimer's, then that means you are probably also of a certain age, and so you might think that I'm giving you a free pass when it comes to the above advice about feeling tired. You might think that, but take me, for example: I'm eighty-four and I go out every single night. Now, I'm lucky that my health allows me to do this, and if you have serious health issues of your own to deal with in addition to taking care of a sick spouse, then I would say your feelings of tiredness are not psychological, but actually physical. But if you're basically healthy, then your tiredness might be a symptom of boredom, and so I want you to find ways to push those types of tired feelings aside.

By the way, while I wrote this section about "tiredness," long before I interviewed any experts in the field, I was later gratified to learn that experts agree with what I believe. The only way to refresh your mind and body when you're a caregiver is by pursuing other interests. If you keep your mind refreshed, then your body will follow suit. But if you let yourself fall into a mental rut, then your overall view of life will change for the worse.

In addition to "feeling" tired, you may also actually be physically tired. If your care recipient keeps you up at night so that you're not getting enough sleep, you may be walking around exhausted. That has many negative effects, including psychological ones. It's easy to make poor decisions when you're overtired. Advice on how to get enough rest doesn't belong in this chapter, but please be aware that if you are sleep deprived, you will encounter psychological effects and your emotions may become amplified. Instead of feeling a little sad when something upsetting happens, you'll feel very sad.

The bottom line is, if you're feeling tired because you're not getting enough sleep or the physicality of being a caregiver is more than your body can take, do what you need to do to get more truly refreshing rest. But, if your feelings of tiredness are really psychological, accept that you're probably bored and do something about that. Whatever the case, be proactive at protecting the health or your body and mind.

Fear

Most of the caregivers reading this book are close relatives to the patient. And, since we know that Alzheimer's has a genetic component, those of you who share the same genes, as opposed to a spouse or in-law, cannot help but wonder whether you may one day wind up in similar circumstances to the person for whom you are caring. Undoubtedly, that thought will leave you fearful. (At the moment, ten genes have been identified that are linked to Alzheimer's, though it is thought when all is said and done the number will be closer to one hundred.) This fear may increase if you are one of those people who reads up on the latest information about any medical condition. I spoke to one person who told me that the children of his great aunt who has Alzheimer's rarely come to visit because there are others in the family who have come down with this disease, and seeing their mother causes them to feel terrified about their own risk. It's a sad situation, but one that's more common than you would think.

Have you ever gone to see a doctor who seemed quite unsympathetic? Part of the reason for that is that doctors couldn't function if they were psychologically exhausted from giving in to too much empathy. A so-called "bedside manner" is important to a patient's healing, but not everyone who goes into medicine can cope as well with seeing people suffering day after day as others can. Some just have to steel themselves against such emotions to get through the day.

Throughout this chapter I've been telling you that it's important to feel your emotions in order to allow yourself to better handle your full range of emotions. But as is often the case, there's an old saying that covers many situations, and the one that applies here: There's an exception to every rule.

Allowing yourself to feel fear can paralyze you. Fear is very hard to push aside once it has a grip on you. If you feel sad and you have a good cry, you can then figure out how to raise your spirits. But fear saps the very thing you need to overcome it—your courage. Fear can paralyze you and leave you helpless. So, if you look at your care recipient and allow yourself to start thinking, "This could be me in twenty years," that type of thinking is just not going to be helpful.

Most importantly, your fears may not be justified. Just because someone close to you develops Alzheimer's doesn't guarantee that you will. And the medical world is starting to make advances with regards to this disease, so even if your genes do include those linked to Alzheimer's, that doesn't mean you will actually fall victim to this disease. So while it may be natural to have such thoughts, my advice is to shove them aside the moment they arise. (The latest thinking is that in people who have a gene that will lead to Alzheimer's, drug treatment should start fifteen years before any symptoms arise. These drugs aren't fully developed yet, but they will be able to prevent damage, not restore damaged tissue, which is why treatment would have to start so early. I understand that no one wants to hear that they have a genetic predisposition to something like Alzheimer's, but it would be so much better to face that fear and be tested on, say, your fortieth birthday than to allow this fear to paralyze you and then later have an incurable case of Alzheimer's.)

Another set of fears that you may encounter can arise from reading about all the problems that accompany dementia. Now, it's good to be prepared. Many of the behaviors associated with advanced Alzheimer's develop slowly, so understanding what you are noticing and being able to deal with it is important. But remember, not every person with dementia develops every one of these behaviors. So there's no point getting yourself all worked up over what might happen when it may never happen.

This role you've taken on is very stressful, and you have to do what you need to do to minimize your level of stress. Thus, if knowing too much will cause you to panic, then don't feel obligated to know more than what you have to. If you're the type of person who does tend to fret, don't spend hours reading up on every little aspect of Alzheimer's. If you notice a new pattern of behavior, such as your mother accusing you of stealing her belongings, that's when it would be appropriate to determine what needs to be done. Maybe you can assign that task to someone else so that you don't get swept up into reading too much about every detail of this disease. Let this other person condense the advice on how to handle this particular pattern of behavior, or see your loved one's doctor or a social worker and ask what you should do in response to the new behavior.

You will probably also run into financial fears. The expense of caring for an Alzheimer's patient can be quite considerable, especially in the later stages. The best way to allay that fear is to see a specialist in Elder Law (read more about this in Chapter 12).

Another potential fear is that of no longer being needed. There are care recipients who really need to be institutionalized, but the caregiver is afraid of what will happen to their life when their loved one is taken away. You might think that they would be relieved, but if you've been a caregiver for a number of years, that role can become a defining part of your identity. You may fear that without that role, you'll collapse into a puddle, like that wicked witch in *The Wizard of Oz*.

This is, of course, an irrational fear. First of all, you'll be spending a lot of time going to the facility, so it's not as if your role as a caregiver is over. Also, once you have more freedom, you'll find plenty of ways to use the time. This is a fear that you have to set aside, because if the time has come for your loved one to go to a facility, then that's what should happen.

Shame

If you're walking down the street with your mother, who has Alzheimer's, and she looks a little confused and isn't dressed as well as she used to dress, should you feel ashamed? Of course not, but that doesn't mean that you might not feel some shame. Maybe up until recently she was someone who took great care of her appearance, and now it's a fight just to get her to comb her hair. You know she could use some fresh air, but while walking around the neighborhood with her, you'd prefer not to run into anyone you know. And if you did run into an acquaintance and your mother said something that revealed that her mind was badly deteriorated, even to someone who knew she had Alzheimer's, you probably would feel ashamed.

A number of friends and acquaintances I've spoken to who are caregivers have reported this reaction. They end up missing out on a lot of socialization because of it. Rather than go out to dinner with friends, they prefer to stay home, afraid that their spouse will in some way act inappropriately.

I hate to keep repeating myself, but the initial onset of our emotions is not under our control, so you might not be able to keep yourself from feeling ashamed in this type of situation. But wouldn't it be terrible if dreading that sense of shame kept you from engaging in a range of activities, in effect becoming housebound because of what other people might think? Having a disease is nothing to be ashamed of, even if the person who has the disease shares some of the blame, the way smoking for a lifetime might cause lung cancer. But with Alzheimer's, there is nothing to be ashamed of, even though the person with Alzheimer's may behave in ways that, under normal circumstances, would be considered inappropriate.

If you were pushing around the wheelchair of a soldier who'd been wounded fighting in a war, would you be ashamed? Not in the least—you might even be proud. Well, life is full of battles, and the person for whom you are caring is in a very tough one with a very nasty disease. But just because their mind has abandoned them doesn't take away from everything they've done throughout their lives. It doesn't diminish their accomplishments one iota. Thus, you must keep those wonderful memories constantly at hand. So, yes, you're walking along with someone whose mind isn't intact, but you're also walking with, let's say, someone who was a great schoolteacher for thirty years and a volunteer at her church, the woman who cooked the best meat loaf in town. I want you to use these memories to push aside your shame so that you won't avoid situations that may be a little embarrassing, but instead face them with your own form of courage.

I know a couple who adopted two children from Korea. The first child came over in great shape, but as soon as they saw the second, they knew that something was wrong. They could have sent her back, but they chose to keep her. Now in her twenties, she is severely disabled in many ways, including mentally. If they all go out to a restaurant, she will go up to strangers and do things that are, let's say, unexpected. But that doesn't stop her adoptive parents from taking her places or loving her to death. That's just the way she is. Most people are very understanding and just smile when she comes up to their table and blows out their candles, as she's wont to do. And, considering all the press that Alzheimer's receives, most people will also realize that your mother isn't her normal self and won't think badly of her, or you. Yes, you may find yourself embarrassed from time to time by the actions of your parent or spouse, but don't let that stop you from remaining a part of society. The days of lepers being ostracized from society are long gone, and Alzheimer's isn't contagious.

Certainly don't keep the fact that your loved one has Alzheimer's from family members because you are ashamed of it. First of all, this is something that's very hard to keep from people, so there's really no point trying. But also, you are going to need their help and support, which won't be forthcoming if you deny the truth about your situation. Whether they like it or not, family members have to accept what is happening. That's just part of what being "family" is all about. In tough times, you all have to come together and support each other.

Sadly, I have to admit that outside of your family you will run into people who, out of ignorance, may react negatively toward your loved one who has Alzheimer's. I read of one community where many people objected to having a facility for people with Alzheimer's being built next to a school. Because the facility would be locked, which was intended to protect the patients from wandering off, not to protect the public from the patients, some community members thought that it would be filled with dangerous residents who posed a risk to their children. This is a preposterous idea, but people who are uneducated or misinformed about Alzheimer's may focus on some negative gossip or rumors they have picked up and then act inappropriately. If you run into such people, try not to be ashamed for your care recipient or to become upset. Just tell yourself that while these people may not be suffering from dementia now, if it ever happens to them they'll have less to forget because they never knew all that much in the first place.

Perhaps the worst thing shame can do to a caregiver is to keep that person from joining a support group. A support group offers caregivers so much, and since everyone who attends these meetings is in the same boat, you just have to push past any shame you might have that could keep you from using that support in the first place. Part of your shame might be that you need help from others, that you're ashamed that you can't do it all. But the truth is that you do need help, and once you start going to a support group, you'll wish you would have gone earlier.

I have a doctor friend whose wife has Alzheimer's. He's not only a doctor, he's also a noted researcher. He's joined two support groups and praises them both. If someone with his credentials isn't ashamed to seek the help of a support group, you shouldn't let shame stop you either.

BITTERNESS

Just because of my family's religion, the Nazis killed all of them. I certainly was bitter toward Germany for many years, but today I go there frequently and was recently the Grand Marshal of the Steuben Day Parade, a German-American celebration in New York.

It's easy to feel bitter when someone you love, who certainly doesn't deserve to have a serious affliction, comes down with one. One can also feel bitter about having to bear the burden of this calamity by becoming the main caregiver. The problem with being bitter is that it makes the situation worse, not better. To wallow in bitterness is a luxury you can't afford. In order for you to make it through every day, you need as much positivity in your life as possible. There are enough external factors that make it tough without you adding to the overall negative atmosphere by being bitter.

What's the opposite of bitterness? Gratefulness. While sadly there are some young people who come down with Alzheimer's, for the most part this is a disease that strikes the elderly. Thus, you have to be thankful for all the wonderful years that this person had, and shared with you, rather than give in to bitterness.

Is it possible to feel grateful regarding something as awful as getting Alzheimer's? My son's father-in-law has Alzheimer's. He caught it early, and the medication he's on is keeping his quality of life, at least for the present, in pretty good shape. He wrote an article for the *Globe and Mail* in Toronto, where he lives, and I'd like to quote from it:

> Sometimes when we are going through hard times, we say, "There's a light at the end of the tunnel." With dementia, I know there is no light. But in many ways my life is growing richer. I notice the colors and textures around me as I walk. I am no longer in a hurry to accomplish things. I have time to delight in my family.
>
> I see my life as a movie, in slow motion where the camera lingers on what is important and often a bright light illuminates a scene. In the amazing mystery of how our brains work, I may not remember what I had for lunch yesterday, but all my early adventures are still within me. I have written many little stories from my life, for my grandchildren.
>
> When my wife took over the driving two years ago, I was at first a constant backseat driver. I have to admit she probably thinks I still am … but I can't believe how pleasant it is now to be a

passenger, gazing at the people and sights as we travel on outings and to our endless appointments.

Robin Leckie isn't grateful for having Alzheimer's, but he is grateful for these final years of his life. He's finding the silver lining in this particular cloud and is making the best of it. I recognize that sometimes it may be hard to feel grateful. Let me compare it to getting exercise. There are going to be many days when you don't want to go to the gym, and there will be lots of excuses to skip going for that jog or bike ride, but in the end, you'll feel better if you do. And so in this case, it's the same thing. If you force yourself to be grateful for all the good rather than be bitter about the bad, in the end you'll be better off.

One way that people exhibit their bitterness, if they are religious, is to put the blame on God. They feel abandoned, they want to know what they did wrong to deserve this, they want God to fix it, and if He doesn't, then He's somehow at fault. Since everyone's religious beliefs are different, I'm not going to go into the area of religion too much, but I also can't ignore it.

Despite all I went through in my life because of my religion, I'm still very religious. I don't think that I have the right to blame God for what men do. Nor do I feel that we have the right to blame God for illnesses. Religion offers we humans much comfort, which is why many people believe in one religion or another. To give up on your religion because of Alzheimer's would be a big mistake, and let's face it, if you are bitter toward God about what has happened, you have given up on your religion. So to me, bitterness of any sort is a losing proposition, and that's especially true in a religious context.

Also, a religious leader, be it a priest, rabbi, imam, or whatever, can be a source of great consolation. He or she has most likely been trained to help people faced with problems such as those you are facing. You will need all the people you can find to lean on, and so if you belong to a religious institution, you need to hold on to your faith so that you will have not only your pastor but the entire congregation helping you to bear the weight you've been given.

One more thing about feelings of bitterness: The more you give in to them, the harder they are to shrug off. My advice to you is that the moment you recognize that you are feeling bitter, think of a reason to feel grateful. When I say "the moment," I mean just that. Don't waste a second on being bitter, because each second will make it harder to shed this destructive emotion.

LONELINESS

You may have spent decades enjoying the companionship of your husband, but today, when he's not making any sense, he's not exactly good company. And, because he needs to be watched all the time, even though you're never physically alone, you could easily end up feeling very lonely yourself.

A close friend of mine whose wife has Alzheimer's reports feeling very lonely for two separate reasons. The first is that because of his wife's condition he doesn't have the opportunity to socialize much. He stays home to take care of her but doesn't feel comfortable being around other people with her, so he's cut off from the outside world to a considerable extent. (This condition is also due, in part, to the fact that he moved from one coast to the other to be closer to his son. This made sense because his son helps him out, but after spending fifty years living in one place, the many friends he and his wife had made are all thousands of miles away.)

The other reason he feels lonely is that he has "lost" his best friend, his wife. He used to be able to talk to her about everything and now he can't. He finds it particularly frustrating that he can't share his emotions with her because she just doesn't understand. (Not being able to read other people's emotions is often something that patients with Alzheimer's struggle with.) So while his natural instinct is to turn to his wife for sympathy, that well is now empty.

He says to himself that after all that he and his wife have shared, he owes it to her to just accept what has happened. He admits to being lonely but feels there is nothing to be done about it. To my way of thinking, his attitude is a mistake, and here's why: Loneliness can reinforce any other negative feelings you may have. It's not easy caring for someone with Alzheimer's, but it's easier if you have friends to lean on for both social and physical support.

In my opinion, you have to find allies to help you fight against the loneliness. The first thing you must do is to tell everyone you know that you welcome company. People might think they're intruding, or they may think that your home has been turned into a hospital ward with limited visiting hours. So, you have to put the word out that your door is always open. Make sure you stock up on some cookies or crackers and cheese or other snacks so that if someone does drop by, you're prepared. More importantly, your attitude has to be welcoming. You have to put a smile on your face even if you don't feel like it, because after spending some time with a sympathetic human being, you will.

Though in-person visits are best at combating loneliness, these days there are a myriad of other ways to connect, and you should use them all. If you have a computer, make sure that you have the ability and equipment to make videophone calls. They're so easy, and free, and having a face to look at will make a phone call seem more like an in-person visit. If a friend or family member isn't available, you can always find people willing to chat on certain sites that feature video. Just be careful not to reveal anything too personal about yourself, and use good common sense.

I know that today people are writing shorter and shorter messages (even I'm on Twitter), but if you're feeling lonely, you may need to say more than you can put in a few sentences. In the old days when people would write letters, they didn't necessarily write them all in one fell swoop but would leave them on their desk and go back to them during the course of the day before mailing them. This allowed them to carry on this conversation in their head, as they thought of things they wanted to put in the letter. Maybe you should do the same thing. Instead of going straight to your e-mail, open up a document in your word processor and take the time to compose an actual letter. Make sure to reread what you write so that you don't leave anything out. Then, when you're ready to send it, cut and paste it into your e-mail program and send it off. Of course, if you don't have a computer, everyone still enjoys receiving a handwritten letter.

As I mentioned before, support groups can be a valuable resource. I'll have more to say about them later in the book, but in addition to allowing members to share information, they also provide company, so use them as a way to connect to other people, even if you don't feel the need to share your personal situation. In fact, at most meetings for caregivers you don't have to say very much about your situation at all. Everyone else in the room is going through a similar situation to yours, so they'll understand if you want to maintain some privacy. But just being among them and listening will make you feel less lonely, and, at some point, you may find that you'll be able to contribute to the conversation.

Finally, don't turn to the television as a companion, because it's not one. There's nothing wrong with watching some TV, but turning on the TV every time you feel lonely will not help your situation. Instead, make an effort to connect with someone in person, or, if that's not an option, via one of the other mediums mentioned above.

GRIEF

Normally, we grieve for someone after they've passed away, but with some medical conditions, when there is no hope for a recovery, we can be overcome with grief even while the afflicted person is very much alive. Alzheimer's patients go through various stages, and you can be filled with grief at any one or even all of them.

In the early stages, when your mother is going in and out of lucidity, sometimes seeming like her old self and at other times showing how much her mental state has diminished, you might begin to grieve the loss of the person you knew. While in the later stages, when you know the end is near, you'll begin to grieve for the coming physical loss.

The length of time that Alzheimer's can affect a person is what makes grief so difficult to deal with. It's one thing to grieve for someone who has died. This is something we've all gone through, and will likely go through again and again in our lives. But how do you grieve for someone who is still living?

Studies have shown that most people who have lost a significant other grieve for about six months. At the end of that period, they begin to go back to a sort of normalcy. (Obviously grief affects everyone differently, but such statistics can serve as useful guidelines sometimes.) Grieving for long periods of time—the years it can take for someone with Alzheimer's to reach the end—is going to wear you down. It will make it much more difficult to give adequate care. Since your attitude as caregiver can be felt by your care recipient, it's important not to be in mourning for the entire time that this person is in your care.

There's no question that seeing the personality of someone you love disappear before your eyes is sad. But try not to allow yourself to begin to grieve until the end of the process. Try to keep your spirits up by concentrating on the good times, both in the past and present, for your sake and that of your care recipient.

DEPRESSION

So far I've been writing about feelings in the so-called "normal range," but sometimes emotions can get out of hand, especially with sadness. When that happens, you go from being sad to being depressed. Depression is quite serious and can affect your overall health. When you're responsible for taking care of someone else, being depressed is even more serious because depression saps your will to be active, yet you need to be an active caregiver. Depression among caregivers is very common. I don't like to cite statistics, because I don't want anyone to become depressed only because they think it comes with the territory, but the numbers are significant. If you're depressed, you need professional help. You may need a prescription of some sort, and only a medical doctor can help you with that.

One sign of depression is feeling very lethargic and sleeping more than would be normal, but that's a luxury you might not have. (In fact, you might even be sleep-deprived.) Other potential signs of depression may include sleeplessness, the inability to experience pleasure, and problems with appetite.

However, depression isn't a condition where you have one major symptom, like the pain of a sore throat. So how can you determine if you are depressed? In my opinion, the key is to talk about the possibility with a caring friend or relative. Tell them how you're feeling and see what they have to say. It's hard for you to be objective when you're in a very stressful situation, which is why a second opinion could be very valuable. If this person thinks that you might be depressed, it's time to see a doctor. Only a medical doctor can make an actual diagnosis, and if you are clinically depressed, then only a doctor can offer you the help you need.

I'd like to add two more important points about depression. The first is that depression often leads to other problems, such as alcoholism, so you need to be aware of that. The second point is that many caregivers who end up having their care receiver sent to a facility become increasingly depressed, so if you're experiencing this situation, please strongly consider seeking professional help.

FRUSTRATION

If there is one emotion that I can guarantee you're going to feel while caring for someone with Alzheimer's, it's frustration. As the disease progresses, your loved one is going to be doing the same things over and over, such as asking you a question that you answered five minutes earlier, and it's going to be very difficult not to become frustrated when this happens. There will be days when such behavior will be easier to handle than others, but I can predict that no matter how sweet and nice a person you are, there are going to be times when you're going to say to yourself, "I can't take this anymore."

Frustration can lead to anger if you let it. That's especially true if you have a tendency toward having a short fuse. However, allowing yourself to get angry at a situation that you can't change is counterproductive. So, how do you keep yourself from feeling frustrated?

Frustration in such cases comes from having a narrow focus. The more you focus on a particular behavior that your care recipient is exhibiting at the present, the more frustrated you are going to be. What you have to do is pull back, much like a movie camera can go from a tight zoom to a shot that takes a wider view. And, just like a movie camera, it's not something that you want to do too quickly, but rather in a slow, deliberate manner.

So let's say your mother has asked you for the fifth time in the last fifteen minutes when dinner will be ready, but it's only three in the afternoon. You've told her each time that it won't be ready for three more hours, but you know from experience that she's going to ask you again any minute and you're going to have a hard time not screaming because you're getting frustrated, especially as various scenes like this play out all day long. So how do you widen the scope for yourself? (In a later chapter, I'm going to give you some advice with regards to helping your care recipient, but here we're talking about your own state of mind.)

What I would advise in this case is to recall some of your favorite memories about food. If appropriate, mention what you're thinking about to your mom. If not, then keep the thoughts to yourself, but rather than focus on the answer you give to her, focus on these memories. Replay the scenes in your head and try to enjoy them as much as you can.

Here I've focused on one example, but obviously there are going to be other similar situations that you'll find yourself in, and the trick is to go in prepared. When I'm feeling blue, for example, I reach into this box of letters I keep that always brings a smile to my face. You may have to spend some time and effort preparing particular paths of memories that evoke pleasant feelings for you. But doing your homework is key. You know what makes you frustrated, so only you can prepare for those moments. And if you do a good job, you'll find that you can greatly reduce those feelings of frustration.

Of course, in the case of repetitive behavior, the best solution would be if you could stop it, so let me offer you some advice for doing that. The first thing you must do is to make sure that your loved one actually understands your answer. If, when you say dinner will be in three hours, she doesn't comprehend the meaning of what you're saying, the message is not going to sink in. See if you can find a method of communicating the thought that she will understand. Let's say she can still read a clock. Get one of those cardboard clocks used to teach children how to tell time, set it to 5 p.m. and show it to her. That might get the message through easier than words. Each person with Alzheimer's loses different abilities at different stages, so you'll have to do some experimenting to figure out what methods of communications might still work.

You must also keep in mind that questions may give you hints of what's going on in her mind. Think whether you can identify a cause for a particular line of questions. For example, if she's asking about dinner, it may indicate that she's hungry, so by giving her a snack, she's likely to stop asking about dinner.

You may also be able to distract your care recipient with another activity, which will stop the flow of a repetitive question. Maybe put on a favorite video. Or give him something tactile to do, like a pile of large Legos to stack together. Again, you might have to experiment a bit to discover which tactile objects will work best. (Many children's toys can work, but there are also products designed especially for those with dementia.)

NEGATIVITY

To a great degree, many of the negative emotions I've been writing about are connected, like frustration leading to anger. Certainly, if you are dealing with a range of negative emotions, your overall outlook can become negative. The subtle difference with negativity is that rather than being an emotion that crops up from time to time, reacting to a specific stimulus, negativity can become a part of your personality that infects everything you do. And a negative attitude can lead to a vicious cycle, because if you start out thinking that you will fail, then it becomes more likely that you will fail.

The most important trick in combating negativity is recognizing it. Once you realize that you are always being negative, you can try to change your attitude. But as long as you're unaware of this cloud over your head, it will continue to affect you, making you miserable.

Negativity is like a trap, always ready to grab your ankles and hold you back. Thus, you have to learn to look around and see where those negativity traps lie and avoid them. For example, if something goes wrong during the day—you burn dinner, for example, because your mom had you busy looking for her hairbrush—you might say, "Oh, these things always happen to me." While you might not have burned dinner in ten years, if you take the attitude that bad things like this happen to you, then they will.

I am not saying that you shouldn't get upset because you burned dinner. I give you five minutes to rant and rave a bit while you clean up and start all over. But after those five minutes are up, take a deep breath or two and move on. Put on some lively music. Forget making dinner and order pizza. Put a portable timer on your shopping list that you can carry with you, so if you're out of the kitchen, you can still keep track of time. By doing a few positive things, you can change your attitude and not be brought down into the dumps because of one thing you did wrong, when overall you're doing a very positive thing—taking care of someone who needs you.

PHYSICAL SIGNS

I've told you to try to be aware of when you're feeling frustrated or negative, and one way of doing that is by becoming aware of physical signs of stress such as shortness of breath, chest pains, or having a knot in your stomach. If your emotions are causing physical symptoms such as these, then you must take action.

First of all, don't hide how you're feeling. Let your other relatives know how much pressure you are under, and hopefully they'll volunteer to give you more breaks.

Often, physical signs of stress can be combated. If you feel short of breath, then stop for a few minutes and take some deep breaths. If you're feeling stressed, try to do some form of exercise, even if it's just walking around the dining room table ten times, though if you can go for a walk outside, all the better.

If you can't shake the physical symptoms of stress on your own, then see your doctor. I'm not a big fan of taking pharmaceuticals, but these manifestations of stress, as well as the unique mental health concerns of your situation, can be quite debilitating, and you need to be careful about your health as you have quite a responsibility being a caregiver.

Your Environment

Your environment has a lot to do with the way you feel. Light, for example, can play a big role, so try to maximize the amount of light in your surroundings. (On the other hand, when trying to communicate with someone with dementia, it can be helpful to keep distractions to a minimum, so closing the curtains might be called for when you're trying to get through to them.) It's great to get out, but if you find yourself stuck indoors a lot, especially in bad weather months, a lamp that simulates daylight can lift your mood. This might be good for the person you're caring for, as well.

I wrote a book entitled *Musically Speaking*. In it, I wrote about the role music played in my life. I've already mentioned how I led the children on the train taking us out of Nazi Germany in song, but though I can't carry a tune, music has always been important to me, and it should be to you, too. Having the right music playing can really lift your mood, as well as that of the person you're caring for. I like classical music best but whatever the style, if it's up-tempo and bright, it will lift your mood. However, if your favorite type of music is dreary, then it is better not to listen to any music because that type of music can make you feel worse.

Color also can play a role when it comes to mood. Bright colors are certainly better than dark ones, and if the person you're taking care of always is partial to a particular color, painting the room they sleep in that color might make their outlook brighter.

I'm not an expert in aromatherapy, but hospitals and nursing homes have found that having the right aromas in the air helps their patients, so I would suggest you look into it. In addition to incense and the like, if you cook in a crock pot, the smell of a nice stew or soup can fill the house for hours. And, whether or not they're fragrant, flowers in a room lift everyone's mood, so whenever you can, keep a bouquet or two around the house.

Then there are pictures. Hopefully, you already know that while patients with Alzheimer's have a big problem with short-term memory, they often can remember the past. So having lots of pictures around of happy times from the past will not only help their mood, but will help you to remember why you're investing so much of your life in taking care of this person.

Finally, in terms of environment, let's not forget temperature. Older people tend to be more sensitive to cold and heat, so you may have to keep your environment at a temperature that doesn't really suit you. Of course, there are ways to accommodate each of you. Making sure your loved one is wearing warmer clothes might allow you to keep the temperature down. The use of a space heater, provided it wouldn't be dangerous to your care recipient, would allow you to heat just a certain portion of a room.

WORKING WITH A PROFESSIONAL

I want to discuss how a professional can help with feelings. Let me start by giving you an example. Let's say that you needed to lose weight. You're at a friend's house and you're offered some cake. You say, "No thanks, I'm trying to lose some weight," but this friend is under several types of pressure to insist. First of all, she planned ahead and bought or made this cake. Then, most societies put great store in being hospitable, which includes offering treats. Finally, she may want some cake, and so she needs you to have some with her so that she doesn't feel like a glutton eating cake all by herself. It's hard to say no, especially if you'd really enjoy having some cake, and you're likely to allow your arm to be twisted and have a piece, right? But what if you were to say, "Sorry, my blood sugar is a little high and my doctor said I can't have any cake." In all likelihood, your host is going to stop trying to pressure you because now you are under doctor's orders.

So now let's consider the decision to send your relative to a facility of some sort. Say you've decided to send your husband to a facility, but your children are pushing back, saying he would be better off at home, where you would continue to take care of him. Even without such pressure you're going to undergo some inner conflict about this decision because you're going to feel guilty. But if you've engaged a professional, a doctor or a social worker, and you can say that this person is recommending sending your care recipient to a facility, this ally will make it a lot easier for you to make this decision, with regards to yourself and your family. Of course, you want the best care for the person with Alzheimer's, but let's be honest, at the present time there is no cure. You need to find someone who will be looking out for you, the primary caregiver, just as much as the patient. If this person knows you, has seen all the effort you've put in, and can tell that you're now at a breaking point, they'll be able to help you make the right decision.

You don't need me to tell you how difficult it can be to be the main caregiver of someone with Alzheimer's. But you do need me to tell you that this is a burden that must be shared to whatever degree is possible. I don't like placing labels on people. It's tempting to say that you're a victim of Alzheimer's, too, but that's beyond the point. What is important is to recognize when you need help, and sometimes that is not a realization that you can make alone.

While I'm going to get into this issue in more depth later, when it comes to sending someone with Alzheimer's to a facility, there really is very little justification for assuming the burden of guilt. That's because being in the company of other people with Alzheimer's can actually be more pleasing to your loved one and offer them a better lifestyle than staying at home with you.

3

You Get to Have a Life, Too

I don't want to appear glib with the title of this chapter. I fully understand that each caregiver's circumstances are different. In one case you might have a daughter taking care of her mother, but she has three siblings who live nearby and can help out, while in another case you have a wife taking care of her husband, without relatives nearby. So in each case, the "life" that I want you to have is going to be different. But my overall point remains the same: that to whatever degree possible, every caregiver must think of him or herself as well as the person who is in their care.

Alzheimer's is a terrible disease, but it mustn't claim two victims. As a caregiver, you do give up a lot, but you don't have to give up everything. If you do, you and your care recipient will end up paying the price because if you push yourself too much, if you don't allow yourself some time off, you just won't have the strength—emotional, psychological, and physical—to keep up your part. You'll fall victim to what's been dubbed "Caregiver Burnout."

Caregiver Burnout is not just a phrase but something that experts in the field see all the time. Sometimes the symptoms are physical, but more often they're mental, with depression being a common one. If you're lucky, the doctor overseeing your care recipient will also be asking you questions and making sure that you're not succumbing to Caregiver Burnout. If this is not the case, then you have to be alert for ways in which you've changed since taking on these duties and seek additional help if you need it.

Let me illustrate the negative effect Caregiver Burnout has on patient care with one example. Often people with mid- or late-stage dementia become argumentative. Since they're not in their right mind, you can't reason with them. Instead, you have to keep a smile on your face and try to divert them from whatever subject they're arguing about. That's not an easy thing to do at any time, but it will be almost impossible if your nerves are badly frayed. Thus, you need to take care of your own needs as much as possible so that you can give the best care possible.

Don't try to manage everything entirely on your own. I've already written about getting family to help, but outside help is also probably available, even in these times of budget cuts. Many localities have agencies that can send someone to your home to give you assistance. On the NeedyMeds website alone (www.needymeds.org/free_clinics.taf), you'll find a list of over 11,000 clinics that offer either free or low-cost help. (For more resources, see the Appendix.) But to get help you have to accept the fact that you need all the help you can get. In making that decision, always bear in mind that if you wind up with burnout, you'll be unable to care for your loved one.

Before I go any further, I know that not everyone reading this book is computer literate and that not everyone has a computer. That's particularly true of seniors, like me. (I rely on my co-author Pierre to do all my research on the Internet.) While this situation presents an obstacle, it's certainly not an impossible one to overcome. There's probably somebody you know—a relative, neighbor, or friend—who can help you do this type of research, and if not, then there are many other places to turn, such as your public library, the office staff of your place of worship, or a social worker at a nearby hospital. You could potentially even hire a local teen who has a computer and could help you out for a modest sum. In fact, if you called a local high school or college, you might even get some young person to volunteer.

Permit me to expand on this last little nugget of advice I just gave because it illustrates the overall point I am trying to make in this chapter. It would take a little chutzpah, the Jewish word for being gutsy, to start calling local schools in a search to find a teen who would volunteer to help you out. In a sense, it would seem like asking for charity for yourself, and that's a little embarrassing. Also, it might take quite a few phone calls before you find the right person to assist you. Or you might make twenty-five calls, only to discover that this particular road was a dead end. Therefore, the most important factor to persuade you to go through a process like this is the belief that you are deserving of this help, that you get to have a life, too. However, if your belief is halfhearted, you are not likely to succeed.

Bear in mind that I've given you a very specific example, but there are actually many ways of finding someone to help you navigate the Internet. I present more about support groups in Chapter 10, but you should definitely become an active member of one, and raising this issue with that group will certainly lead you in the right direction, which might not be a local high school at all. But I do know that there are high schools that make a commitment to help older citizens in the community, so it's possible that even if you were searching blindly, without any guidance, your search would lead you to a volunteer.

I wish I had the time to take each one of you by the hand and guide you through your life to make it better. Since I don't, I wrote this book, offering you my general advice, and helping you to believe that your need to have a life is a very important part of what I have to offer. When I say "believe," I don't just mean for you to say "I get it" and put it out of your mind. I mean for you to take an active role in making sure that you do what it takes to give yourself as much of a life as possible.

But There's No Time

How many of you said that to yourself as you read the title to this section? As I said, each of you has different circumstances, so statements like, "Of course, there's time" will mean something different to each of you. But while I can't tell you exactly how much time is available to you, I can do something else: I can help you to figure out how to spend your time. I want you to write down how you spend your time over the course of the next two or three days so that you get a typical breakdown of each day. Write down everything you do and how long it takes. Then be honest with yourself and analyze where you could carve out the time for something as important as making a life for yourself. I bet there are plenty of windows of opportunity, though maybe you'll have to be a little creative.

Here's an example of what I mean by being creative: Let's say it takes you half an hour to prepare dinner each night. On the one hand, you're busy, but it's also a task that doesn't take up all of your attention. You might spend the extra time the cooking process allows by talking on the phone with a friend. But since you need your hands to cook, you might need some simple equipment, like a speakerphone, or a portable or cell phone that would allow you to plug a little headset into it so you could stick the phone in your pocket and have both hands free to prepare the meal. If you did that, suddenly the time you use for one job could also be used to do something for yourself, like catching up with a friend. There are other things that you could do while cooking. You could listen to music. You could listen to a book on tape. You could listen to the news, or, if you have a small TV in the kitchen, watch your favorite show.

So, first, spend several days keeping this diary in order to identify where you might make some time for yourself. You'll also need to spot blocks of time on your list that may appear to be full, but that actually offer the potential for you to add some extra pleasure to them. Then you have to figure out how to make it all work. Yes, it will take some effort; let me reiterate that you can find the time to improve the quality of your life, but you have to have the incentive to do so. To have that incentive, you have to truly believe that you are deserving of a life.

Now why might you not believe that? The biggest reason is that you have this burden. After a while, the responsibilities of taking care of someone who requires so much of your time and energy can sap you of resources. The days pile up and the entire process starts to overwhelm you. As your energy drains away, you start to forget that you're "you" and not just a caregiver. Your sense of worth begins to evaporate and your self-esteem begins to spiral downward. It's not surprising that you could become overwhelmed by your situation. But understand, it doesn't have to be this way.

I'm sure you know the word "momentum." People who follow sports are probably the most familiar with it because if you watch football or basketball games, you will often witness how a single play can change the momentum of the game, so that the team that seemed to be losing badly suddenly turns everything around and catches up. If your life is spiraling downward, your job is to break the momentum of that spiral so that you can start improving things. Just like with sporting events, it doesn't have to take much to get things going in the right direction.

Let's say that you placed an announcement in the bulletin of your house of worship that you were looking for someone to volunteer a few hours a week to help you take care of your husband, who has Alzheimer's. And, let's say that one of the members of the congregation, a high school student looking to bolster her applications for college with some volunteer activities, calls you up and offers her services. Suddenly, for two afternoons a week, you'll have a cheery young person around brightening up the place. And, while she takes your husband out for a walk, you'll be free to do something that you really want to be doing. (Whatever you do, don't use this free time for chores. Remember, this chapter is about making your life better.)

Of course, you could place that ad and receive no response at all. Here's my philosophy about that. My favorite animal is the turtle. I actually have hundreds of them. None are real, but once word got out that I like turtles, people started giving me little turtles made out of this or that material. In any case, the reason I like turtles is because they're living proof that if you want to get anywhere, you have to stick your neck out. A turtle is safe when tucked inside its shell, but in order to live, it has to move about. I see one of my jobs in life as getting people to break out of their shells and take risks. While there are no guarantees when you take a risk, there's also little chance of changing the momentum of your life if you don't.

Here's another key word with regard to this chapter: incentive. In order for you to get up the gumption to take a risk, like calling around looking for a young volunteer, you need a good incentive. For the turtle, it's the need to look for food or a mate. For you, it can't be just to have a few hours to do your chores. Chores need to be done and you'll almost always find the time to do them. They come with their own built-in incentive: necessity. However, engaging in a hobby, reading the latest book by your favorite author, spending an hour at the gym working up a sweat, all these can be put off, and probably often are. One reason may be that you don't feel they're all that important. You look at the things you could do for yourself as luxuries, not necessities. You need to change your attitude so that you'll have the incentive to make the changes in your life that will allow you to obtain the added pleasure I'm advocating.

Just as you need food to keep your physical body going, you need psychic nourishment to replenish your mental energy levels in order to keep everything humming along. That nourishment comes in the form of things that you do for yourself that are pleasurable and stimulating. I've said it before but it bears repeating. I'm not talking about watching TV or reading a trashy novel. I'm not saying these activities are off-limits, but they're like junk food. They may be tasty at the time you enjoy them, but they don't provide you with the nourishment you need. They're full of empty calories.

What I want you to do is to exercise your mind. In the same way exercise makes your body stronger, exercising your brain makes your mental state stronger. And the stronger your mental state, the better you'll be able to cope with all that you face on a day-to-day basis. Taking care of someone with dementia saps your psychic energy. You need to find ways to improve your ability to cope with this burden and not allow it to force you into being its slave. You have to become stronger, and the only way to do that is to make the time to do things that will give you the mental and psychological strength you need.

Let me offer another example: puzzles. There are word-hunting puzzles where you stare at the page trying to find the words that are hidden among the letters. Mindless. Then there are crossword puzzles where you really have to think in order to find the answers. They force you to use your brain, and by exercising your brain you make it stronger, and this helps you to be more resistant to the rigors of caring for someone with Alzheimer's.

For some of you, what I'm recommending is going to pose quite a challenge, and I understand that. You might find that the path of least resistance is to keep playing the martyr, to suffer through every day, complaining bitterly about your terrible burden. My suggestions are certainly not going to remove that burden. But let's put an image on that burden. Let's say that for your job, you were forced to strap a thirty-pound weight to your back. At the end of the day, when you finally got home, the path of least resistance would be to say, "I'm exhausted" and lie down. However, if you did that, the next day would be just as hard. But if instead you went to the gym and developed stronger muscles, after a time those thirty pounds would seem much lighter.

Like with physical exercise, you have to do this intellectual "something for yourself" regularly. A doctor friend told me that he makes sure to do one thing for himself every day. The path of least resistance might be to put off doing this one thing for yourself, so you have to make a routine out of it. People who go to the gym regularly often have a hard time getting out the door of the gym following a workout, but they're always glad they did when they get back home. You, too, may need to put some extra effort into doing this one thing for yourself, but you'll also reap the rewards.

For those of you who are saying, "But, Dr. Ruth, life is so hard as it is and you want me to make it even harder," I have this to say: I am not telling you to do something that will make you miserable. If you like to paint, I want you to paint a picture. If you like to sew, I want you to make yourself a new dress. If you like mental challenges, then do a complicated crossword puzzle. Or, go online and play chess against an opponent. The hard part is making the time, not deciding whatever it is you are going to do with this time. Your mind needs variety. If all you are doing is working, your mind will revolt and make life even harder. You have to reward it now and then with some intellectual stimulation.

ASAP

I'm sure there are many people who are going to read the above sections, say to themselves, "Dr. Ruth is right, I have to get a life," and then not do a thing about it. They'll promise themselves that they'll get to it as soon as … well, you fill in the excuse. It's like the diet that you're always starting tomorrow—it never gets anywhere.

Usually, you see the initials ASAP (as soon as possible) stamped on business documents by a boss who wants a job done right away. But you already have so many jobs, there's a good chance that this program to get a life will never get started, which is why I want you to stop dawdling and get to work on it ASAP. I've given you a very simple way to begin. All you need to do is get a piece of paper, a pen, and a watch and begin writing down how you are using your time. If you're making the bed, record how long it takes, and also write down when you do it. Do the same with your entire day, and do this for at least two days, though a day or two more might produce a better indication. Now, how hard is it to do that?

Of course, for this diary to be of use, you have to be both complete and honest. If it appears that you're not really as busy as you thought you were, don't start stretching out how long it takes you to do a task. If you see that you spend two, three, or more hours a day watching TV, don't omit that from your diary, even if you're not proud of it. If it is apparent that your day is not as full as it seemed to be, allow yourself to accept the fact that you have been wasting time and promise yourself that from now on you're going to figure out how to put those precious minutes and hours to better use. If those days with empty stretches seemed interminable, remember that it was in part because any time you wasted on doing something mindless wasn't really satisfying. You'll discover that when you're using that time to do something really interesting, your days will seem to move by much quicker.

Of course, if you really have been very busy, and empty slots of time are just not that obvious, the next step will be to examine this diary, looking for holes where you could substitute activities that you could be doing for yourself. Again, this is not a major chore I'm urging you to do. It will probably take you less than half an hour and you might even find it fascinating. Remember, there is nothing on this earth more precious than the time we have here, as it's ultimately limited. So looking at how you use your time and figuring out how to maximize its use ... well, it's like the opposite of paying bills, because every second you retrieve from the waste pile goes right into your pocket.

ALONE TIME AND TOGETHER TIME

I don't want to leave the impression that time for yourself necessarily means time away from the person who is under your care. If you enjoy some outdoor physical activity, like running or playing tennis, then yes, you can't do that with your care recipient at your side. But let's say you greatly admire Impressionist paintings; you could look at a book filled with the paintings of Monet and Cézanne together with the person under your care. Depending on what stage of Alzheimer's your care recipient has reached, you might even be able to visit a museum together. (I saw a PBS special that showed how important art can be to people with Alzheimer's. Yes, they've lost many mental abilities, but it seems that part of the brain that appreciates art remains intact, so looking at art might be a pastime that you can still share.)

As I've said, you're going to need to exercise some creativity to carve out time for yourself, and in order to do that you may have to figure out ways of doing things for yourself while you're also watching over your mother or father. If a particular activity also gives them pleasure, that's wonderful and you'll be able to share the experience, even if your reaction to the experience is a little different than theirs.

By the way, I've put down TV-watching a fair number of times already, but characterizing watching TV as a waste of time is really only true if you're watching commercial television. There are certainly some wonderful, educational, stimulating shows on public television. You can also rent programs that are quite educational and designed to teach you some subject. The person you're caring for perhaps won't understand what you are watching, but there's every chance he or she doesn't understand what's going on if you're watching a silly sitcom either. But having you in the same room, and having some stimulation coming from the TV, may be quite satisfying in and of itself.

Of course, these days there is so much information to soak up from the Internet. If you have a tablet (like an iPad) or laptop, you can be sitting right next to your father and still be connected. You can even take courses that way. It's also possible to have what is on your computer shown on a large screen TV. That way, you can move around, do something useful like help your father to eat his lunch, and also keep an eye on the TV, which is offering your brain some nourishment.

How much your care recipient understands of all this will depend at what stage she is. Let's say you were watching a show that was teaching you how to sketch. Your mother might not fully understand what is being said, but the demonstrations taking place on screen might give her a lot of pleasure. Or, if you have an audiobook playing in the background, she may not fully be able to understand the story, forgetting what happened a few moments ago, but she might still appreciate hearing the stream of words. You have to experiment a bit. If your care recipient becomes nervous and upset when an audiobook is played aloud, then that activity won't be possible to do together. But it might be possible for you to sit there with your mother, stroking her hair or gently rocking with your arm around her while listening to a book via an iPod in your pocket and an earphone in one ear. Many people with dementia take great comfort having someone near them, but you don't necessarily have to be fully involved when you are with them; you just have to be there.

Of course, any plans you have made to take part in activities together may wind up being altered at the last minute if there is a change in your care recipient's mental or physical state. So, while I would encourage you to try to engage in some activities that fulfill your needs together, you still need to find moments when you can do things by yourself so that your enjoyment isn't always hanging by a thread. Again, the more you can do for yourself, the more you will be able to do for the person for whom you're caring—and so you'll actually be doing both of you a favor.

Going to Work

You might not think of going to work as an activity you do for yourself, but it can be. First of all, I would hope you get some satisfaction from doing your job, whatever it is. If you work with other people, going to work can be a good opportunity to socialize. I'd say even if all you made, financially speaking, was just enough to cover the costs of transportation and paying someone to look after your care recipient, keeping your day job might be well worth it. My doctor friend wanted to retire to take care of his wife and I talked him out of it. He's very grateful to me for doing so.

If you're retired, assuming you can find the time or money to hire a replacement for yourself, volunteering outside of your home could be a good substitute. Let's say that your local school needs volunteers to tutor children after school hours. Being around some young people two or three afternoons a week might really pick up your spirits.

Going to the Doctor

Of course, the most important thing you can do for yourself is to take care of your own health. Every report on caregivers shows that most don't do a good job of staying healthy. They'll take the person they're caring for to the doctor but won't go themselves. They literally are putting their lives on the line, because by ignoring symptoms, they end up with serious illnesses. Thus, making sure that you take care of your physical health is priority number one, for your sake, for the person you're taking care of, and probably for the rest of your family, because if you get sick and can no longer act as caregiver, someone else will have to step up to the plate, maybe having now to care for two people.

Saying the phrase "Get a life" to someone can be a pejorative. It's often said to a busybody who is sticking his nose into someone else's business. I hope you understand that I'm not being a busybody myself when I tell you to "Get a life." If I didn't fully appreciate how hard it is to be a caregiver to someone with Alzheimer's before writing this book, I certainly do now. But my research also proved to me how important it is for caregivers not to become completely swallowed up in their role. So, please take some steps, today, to carve out some time for your life, and always remember the importance of caring for yourself and of seeing a doctor regularly to protect your own health.

4

When You're Taking Care of Your Spouse

If you're a caregiver and the person with Alzheimer's is your spouse, the nature of your burden is different. (For those of you whose "spouse" is a gay partner, see more specific information that applies to you at the end of this chapter.) In all likelihood, you've spent decades living side by side. You've been companions, lovers, and, hopefully, even best friends. You've probably shared the duties and joys of parenthood. Your lives are completely intertwined, and now one of you is unraveling right in front of the other.

I always tell couples how important communication is in a relationship, and that advice is even more important to a couple being torn apart by Alzheimer's, at least during the early stages when communication is still possible.

I know that you're both going to be very afraid of the future, and because of that fear, and because talking about the future will raise all sorts of emotions and probably be very sad, you may both avoid the subject, preferring to live for the moment, trying not to spoil whatever pleasure the two of you can have as a couple. I'm not recommending that you talk about your future together all the time. But it is vital that you have at least one in-depth conversation on this subject. Whether or not you can settle every question that is bound to arise in one long talk, you should at least raise all the important issues having to do with finances, institutionalization, and end-of-life matters. At some point, sooner rather than later, I would go one step further and say that the results of this conversation should be written down and signed by both parties. I'm not talking about a legal document, although some legal papers will have to be signed (but those will have to be prepared by a lawyer). No, here I'm talking about the simple agreement the two of you make so that the caregiver and other family members will know, without a doubt, what the spouse with Alzheimer's wished for when he or she remained of sound mind.

I am certain that the spouse headed down the road of Alzheimer's is going to want to ease the burden of his or her partner as much as possible. You both know what's ahead, at least in general terms, and if you love each other, you're not going to want either party to be laden with guilt, but that guilt will surely appear if you don't iron out your future ahead of time.

Denial

Of course, you can't have a heart-to-heart talk about your future if one or both of you are in denial. Not wanting to face the truth is completely understandable, and you don't have to face it on a daily basis while the spouse with Alzheimer's is still in the early stages. But it's also something you can't avoid. I read a blog post from a primary care physician who treated people with Alzheimer's but could not see it developing in his own wife. It was his daughter who made the diagnosis. And, despite his having tried to help his patients cope, he found it very difficult to "walk the walk" for himself.

I know that I can be stubborn, but if enough people, or the right people, tell me I am making a mistake, I listen. When you're in denial about something that you think affects only you, it's possible to drift along for quite a while in that state of denial. But if others are telling you that you are making a mistake and if whatever it is seems obvious to the world and you refuse to listen, then you have to stop yourself. You have to have a heart-to-heart talk with yourself, and then look the problem, whatever it is, in the eye and admit that it is there. Only then will you be able to get the help you obviously (to everyone else) need. Only when you accept the truth will you be able to have an intelligent, rational conversation with your spouse.

Moving Your Spouse to a Facility

Let's start with the hardest topic—making the decision about a facility. As the disease has progressed, you've been taking care of your spouse at home because you want to make sure that he or she is getting the best treatment possible, including your loving touch. But in the later stages of the disease, you might not be able to provide the type of care someone with advanced Alzheimer's requires. In a good facility, people with Alzheimer's will socialize in ways that may be more satisfying than being with you. Also, facilities often provide special classes that will provide stimulation that you can't offer. Even though it may be difficult, put in the effort to find the best available facility, rather than force your loved one to stay home with you if that's not the optimum situation.

If you're older, you're probably having to fight some health battles of your own, making it that much harder to be a caregiver. The burden is going to be a very tough one. Your spouse wouldn't want to see you suffer, especially on their account. That's why it is vital that your spouse gives you permission to be sent to a facility at a certain point before you're over your head with caregiving duties. I'm not saying that you won't feel terrible and racked by guilt, but if your spouse has made you promise that you'll do this, it will be a lot easier to make such a decision knowing that the choice doesn't rest entirely on your shoulders. (Admittedly, I'm ignoring the financial side of this issue, as the costs of being in a good facility may be out of reach for some, which I fully understand.)

If you've been equal partners through life, then you have to be equal partners when it comes to making tough decisions. Of course, if your spouse is already not mentally capable of making decisions, then the decision is yours. But just as most people obey the funeral arrangement wishes of a person who has passed away, you should heed the wishes (if any were expressed) of your spouse if your spouse expressed them while still capable of thinking clearly. The choice to go to a facility is an important example of this. Of course, he or she will never really know whether or not you complied with their wish, as they won't remember it, but that's not the point. The point is that when your spouse was of sound mind, he or she didn't want to see you overburdened by having to handle responsibilities that were more than you could handle.

I understand that you want to continue to take care of a spouse right up until you reach your limits, but once you hit that wall, it's important not to stubbornly resist. You have nothing to feel guilty about, especially if your spouse has given you full permission to find them care outside of your home. Since there's no real reason for you to feel guilty, you needn't suffer.

Will you feel terribly guilty during the first weeks when your spouse is no longer in your care? Most probably you will. Having your loved one in a facility will not relieve you of your burden. In fact, for some people, it is actually worse. But when the time comes when you can no longer offer the care that your loved one needs, you must take this step. You wouldn't try to perform surgery on a sick spouse who required it, would you? Well, if twenty-four-hour special care is required, you must admit that you're not up to that task, either.

Naturally, you'll want to visit as often as possible, though getting there may be quite difficult, particularly if you no longer drive. In deciding which facility to use, ease of access should be an important consideration. But you will also feel very relieved, and you have to tell yourself that no matter how guilty you feel, you actually don't have any reason to feel that way. You did the best you could, and now your spouse is no longer in a state where he or she can stay at home.

Your marriage vows probably included the phrase "in sickness and in health." But Alzheimer's pushes the limits of that vow beyond anyone's endurance. When your spouse's mind and personality are so severely altered, and when tending to their safety, and sometimes even yours, goes beyond your capabilities, it's time to end your duties as a day-to-day caregiver. However, it's helpful to keep in mind that you will continue to oversee your spouse's care in a facility, so you'll still be heavily involved in his or her life.

YOUR CHILDREN

One of the reasons that I advised you to write down and sign the game plan you devise is not just because it will make you, the spouse, more at ease (though it will). Assuming you have children, such a document may play a vital role is keeping family friction to a minimum. If, when the time comes to send your spouse to a facility, one or more of your grown children objects, being able to prove that you are actually carrying out Mom or Dad's wishes can keep the conflict level low.

This is especially true in the case of blended families. If your spouse was divorced, then his or her natural children may feel that they have more say-so than you do. Of course, if you're the one devoting all of your time and energy to caregiving, that's not true. And, even if they really do a fair share of helping, most of the burden is still on your shoulders. Being able to show them a letter signed when your spouse was still of sound mind might avoid, or at least lessen, some nasty arguments.

I'm not one of those in favor of prenuptial agreements, though I can see their utility in some cases. When you marry, it really is in the hopes of being united for life. But Alzheimer's is a unique disease, considering both the severity of the symptoms and the duration of a patient's survival, so being prepared with written instructions just makes good sense, particularly if by doing so you can make the later stages a little less contentious.

YOUR RELATIONSHIP

Retired Supreme Court Justice Sandra Day O'Connor's husband has Alzheimer's and is in a facility where he found a new girlfriend. Justice O'Connor has said she is happy for him, given that he no longer remembers her. It turns out that this is a common occurrence, and it is certainly one of the many oddities of this disease. I bring this up because it illustrates the predicament that you find yourself in. You want to remain faithful, as part of the marriage vow is "til death do us part," but your spouse likely no longer has any idea that your marriage ever took place.

Your wedding anniversary arrives, and with whom do you celebrate it? Is it sadder to drink a toast by yourself or not to mark the occasion at all? Your world is turned upside down because you still have a spouse, and yet at the same time the spouse you knew has vanished.

There is no doubt in my mind that Justice O'Connor has chosen the right attitude. Jealousy has no place in the world of Alzheimer's. But what about the other half of this marriage? Should you be willing to find a new person to fill the void in your life?

Before you answer that question, I want you to separate the rest of the world from yourself. In other words, it doesn't matter what anybody else thinks. The decision to bring someone new into your life while your spouse is still alive is entirely yours. Understandably, the people who are potentially going to have the biggest problem with this are your children, if you have any. Your spouse is their mom or dad, and the idea that you are going to "abandon" your partner probably won't sit well with them. To that, I say, "*C'est la vie*"—that's life. Since there is no way of telling how long your spouse will live—he or she may even outlive you—the changes brought about to your marriage by Alzheimer's shouldn't condemn you to a life of loneliness, and no one, not even your children, should hold it against you.

I'm not saying that finding a new partner is something you should prioritize. But nor is it something you should necessarily avoid. It all depends on what makes you feel best. Though it's not your spouse's fault, you've been abandoned. If you need the companionship, the love, and yes, the sexual gratification of a relationship, then by all means seek one out. You shouldn't have to give up such important assets, especially after all you've gone through, particularly because of other people's opinions.

Sometimes, grown children can be very vocal in their objections. This happens to widows and widowers too, which goes to show you that the children's reaction is far more emotional than rational. There are parents of teens who give up much or all of their sex life because their children are around and they don't feel they have enough privacy. Such parents are giving up way too much of their lives, and their children don't even realize it, and so don't appreciate this "sacrifice." Children—of any age— may be uncomfortable with their parents having sexual needs, but that doesn't mean they have veto power. The same goes for someone in a situation where their spouse is no longer available to them because of Alzheimer's.

I am not saying that anyone whose spouse has some terrible disease that makes it impossible for them to have sex has my permission to go out and have sex with somebody else. Alzheimer's is much different. If someone's brain has changed so that they don't know you exist, and if your potential relationship will have no effect on them and won't cause them any jealousy, then you're entitled to a Get Out Of Jail Free card. But you don't have to use it. That's up to you.

By the way, I know I became famous talking about sex, but the reasoning behind what I'm saying has less to do with sex than fighting loneliness. If your spouse is in a facility and doesn't recognize you when you visit, it may be difficult to continue to consider them your closest companion. No matter what your age, you'll benefit from having some companionship. (If your spouse is much older than you, or if your spouse has early-onset Alzheimer's, that's an even stronger reason to look for a new partner.) The fact that most people spend at least part of their lives in a relationship shows that we have an innate need to form a close bond to someone else. And sex is part of the glue that holds such relationships together. So while perhaps you don't feel a very strong desire for sex (though it's a nice bonus), the fact is, if you want the companionship that comes from a relationship, you probably are going to have to accept the entire package, which will include a sexual component. It's that sexual component that causes everyone around you to become upset, but so be it.

A Change in Status

While your spouse is still alive and possibly still under your care in your home, you're going to face other types of issues as your relationship changes. I have a close friend who is bothered by the fact that his wife no longer recognizes his emotions. It's one of the symptoms of Alzheimer's; the victim loses the ability to "read" people and can no longer understand the subtext of what they're saying via their body language. This loss makes them more gullible and so at risk for being cheated by con artists. But in the case of a husband and wife, when one partner no longer acknowledges the emotions of the other, this changes the dynamics of the relationship in so many ways. And an important aspect of this change is how the healthy spouse feels. If happiness, sadness, anger, fear, and so forth can no longer be communicated, it adds to the healthy spouse's feelings of loneliness.

Another change that slowly develops and impacts the relationship is sharing of responsibilities. Usually, each partner takes responsibility for certain activities in the relationship. But because of Alzheimer's, as the caregiver you're going to have assume responsibility for everything. That's a burden on you, but you usually won't have a choice. This may also cause some conflicts between you and your spouse. For example, if your husband used to do the majority of the driving, at least when you were together, and now he mustn't be allowed behind the wheel of a car, that may make him frustrated and angry. He may take it out on you. What you have to remember is that he's not really mad at you, but he is instead frustrated by the limits being placed upon him by the disease.

Robin Leckie, who wrote that article I quoted earlier, admitted he was a very bad "backseat driver" at first when his wife had to do all the driving. But now he enjoys being relieved of that burden as he can better enjoy the scenery. What this tells you is that to some extent you have to allow time to heal some of these wounds. Yes, your spouse may feel angry at first, and who can blame him, but eventually he'll come to terms with it.

How about your reaction to having to carry the full load? There's no getting around the fact that it's going to be difficult, but the more you fret about it, the worse it will seem. Somehow, you have to dig deep into the well of your love for your spouse, like the parent of a newborn who doesn't want to get up two and three times in the middle of the night but who certainly would never dream of taking it out on the baby. Your spouse is becoming your baby, and emotionally you have to learn to accept that. Since in all likelihood it's going to be long, slow process, try to adapt using a step-at-a-time approach. Staring into the future and fore-seeing all the burdens that lie before you is not going to be helpful.

One of those issues that you may already be facing (but probably lies ahead) is that when you're talking to your spouse, you may not know which spouse you are talking to. Alzheimer's causes delusions. Especially in the early stages, when your spouse is "normal" most of the time, you may not realize for a time that he or she has suddenly gone elsewhere. You'll be hard-pressed to know which husband you're talking to, the one you always knew or the one who's suddenly in another place because of his disease. That is going to frustrate both of you. If you always assume that your spouse is not of sound mind, he or she is going to get very angry at you when not he or she is not delusional, so you have to tread carefully. One thing you can do is not start a serious conversation without knowing the state of your spouse's mind. Start with simple questions that will allow you to judge your spouse's mental acuity and then decide what tack to take.

FIGHTING

Every couple endures fights, some more than others. Because of those fights, you develop certain reflexes. You grow buttons that your spouse knows how to push. Now, however, you find yourself in a situation where your spouse may be doing a lot more button pushing, and yet you can't react in the ways you have previously. It's pointless to get into an argument with someone who is not in full control of his or her mental state. So how do you get through the day?

When I was in the orphanage in Switzerland, one of my duties was to take care of the younger children, and once I immigrated to Palestine,

I studied to be a kindergarten teacher. When I lived in Paris, I taught kindergarten. In this country, I got my doctorate at Columbia Teacher's College. So, I know a thing or two about taking care of young children, and taking care of someone with dementia has certain similarities to tending to young children.

You can't be a cruel kindergarten teacher, because the children will burst into tears. You have to maintain discipline, but you have to do it with a smile, so that your students will want to come to school the next day. The way you do that is by having the day planned out, with lots of spare activities hidden up your sleeve in case one of those you had planned isn't working out quite right. When taking care of someone with Alzheimer's, you have to try a similar strategy. You have to smile even when you want to scream or cry, because your spouse will take cues from your emotional reactions, and if you show that you're upset, your spouse is likely to become upset as well, and the atmosphere will only get worse. You have to keep in mind that words won't always get through as readily as body language.

While it may be hard to mask your emotions, you also have to realize that your emotions can fool you. Under normal circumstances, if you face a problem, you try to fix it. But Alzheimer's can't be fixed. You may feel frustrated and angry, but that's not going to help the situation. You have to learn to accept that your spouse has Alzheimer's, and there's nothing you can do about it but try to make the best of each day, hard as that may be. So, controlling your emotions when your spouse pushes your buttons is practice for doing so at other times, like when you're dealing with repetitive behavior or when your spouse acts inappropriately in front of people. Getting upset isn't going to help the situation. By letting go, by not trying to control something you can't, you'll both be better off.

By the way, I offer some more detailed practical advice for caregivers of all varieties, gathered from various experts, in Chapter Nine. In this chapter, I want to concentrate on the unique situation faced by spouses because your lives are more closely intertwined than other caregiver-care recipient relationships. You deserve this special attention.

SEX

A question faced by every couple affected by Alzheimer's has to do with sex. Whether your partner is in the early stages of Alzheimer's or the latter stages, whether your relationship is still very much together or whether it has been shattered, does it mean that your sex life has to end?

Let me first say that while this topic is not one that is usually covered in materials concerning Alzheimer's, it is an important one, and I'm not the only one saying so. Yes, I speak about sex all the time, but the doctors who tend to patients with dementia all recognize that sex is part of the overall set of problems that couples must face. It was specifically recommended to me by some of these doctors that I cover this area. So, if this has been on your mind, know that you're not alone and that any questions you have are completely legitimate.

Alzheimer's progresses slowly in most cases, and it's not as if you're going to hit the off-switch regarding sex the second you hear a diagnosis of Alzheimer's. First of all, as the caregiver, there's no physical reason for you to give up on sex. You can't do any physical harm to each other. (This can be a concern for couples when one has a heart condition.) But while the sadness that may hang over you upon hearing this diagnosis might inhibit your ability to become aroused, try not to let this happen. Having orgasms release endorphins, which make you feel better, so you shouldn't abandon this source of relief. Additionally, the person with Alzheimer's would feel terrible if he or she was rejected by a spouse because they were in the early stage of this disease. Initially, your sex life can and should continue. But at some point you are going to encounter changes that may put an end to it, and that will be one more aspect of how this terrible disease is going to affect your marriage.

Your sex life as a couple has always been private and that's not going to change. The most important thing I want to say about this subject is not to worry about what society, your children, your neighbors, or the postman would think if they knew you were continuing to have sex or had stopped having sex. This doesn't mean that you must keep having sex through the various stages of this disease, but it also means that there doesn't come a specific time where you should stop. It's a decision that you have to make together.

The fact is that sex feels good, even to someone who has Alzheimer's. If you were both enjoying sex before your lives were turned upside down by this disease, there really is no reason to stop if you still want to have a sexual relationship. And I would encourage you to continue as long as possible—but remember, this isn't my decision, it's yours. If you feel uncomfortable having sex with a spouse who is not all there, then don't.

But if you're sitting on the fence, if you're not sure, then I would urge you to continue.

One reason I'm saying this is that if sex has always been part of your life together, it's important to hold on to whatever remains of the bonds that form your relationship. Let's say you two used to have a cocktail together every evening as you watched the sunset. Unless the doctor has told you that your spouse shouldn't drink alcohol, then I say continue to do so. (And you could always substitute a non-alcoholic drink for your spouse. More about alcohol and Alzheimer's in Chapter Nine.) At some point, your spouse may no longer remember this routine, but you will, and whatever brings you together, even if it's only in your mind, will make it easier for you to get through your day. You need help maintaining awareness that this person is still the same one you married, so sharing special moments together will help you. And, of course, that applies to sharing sex.

By the way, sex or making love doesn't have to follow the same routine as previously. For example, your spouse will definitely enjoy the gentle touch of a nice massage. If you are both nude, and even if only one of you desires sexual satisfaction, in that situation, this can easily be accomplished. You need to acclimate yourselves to what Alzheimer's is doing to your relationship, but that acclimation does not have to mean forced celibacy.

If you need sexual release and your spouse does not want to engage in any sexual interplay, then I would tell you not to hesitate to masturbate.

Some people with Alzheimer's seem to lose their inhibitions, which may mean that your spouse will want more sex than you were used to having before. (Sometimes a hypersexuality comes to the forefront in later stages of Alzheimer's, even if in the prior stages the care recipient showed no interest in sex at all.) Or else, sex may be one of the few pleasurable activities left to him or her, which may also make it more desirable. However, if you were to give in all the time, sex could become one more burden of being a caregiver. My advice in such situations is to say no when you need to, but to also say yes from time to time. You don't want your relationship, your marriage, to turn into merely a nurse/patient one. You are still husband and wife, and having sex can add intimacy that will make your life together less stressful, because the more you drift apart, the harder it will be on you. Of course, in the later stages of the disease, this advice may not apply.

Some people who have Alzheimer's give up on sex. This may be a result of the disease, or it may stem from feelings of depression, especially during the early stages of Alzheimer's when your loved one understands what is happening and what is going to happen. Even if your sex life disappears, don't stop touching one another. The more that verbal skills are lost to the disease, the more other ways of communicating gain in importance, and touch is one way of showing a range of emotions that can be very comforting.

I have read reports that erectile dysfunction (ED) is common among males with advanced Alzheimer's. ED may make having intercourse impossible, though that doesn't mean that you can't still pleasure each other. Do not attempt to give a male care recipient experiencing ED a drug like Viagra without checking with his physician. There could be repercussions if it interfered with any other medications he was taking.

Some wives complain that their spouse who is suffering from ED will blame them for the problem, even though it is not their fault. Of course, people with Alzheimer's tend to blame their caregiver for all sorts of problems, many of which are delusional. Learning to accept such criticism, and trying to deflect it by switching topics while not showing any emotion, especially anger, is one of the talents that caregivers must develop, without letting the stress of such theatrics get to them. I don't know if it is any sadder that something that once gave the two of you so much pleasure—sex—has now become just one more source of stress, but it certainly is not easy, that I understand.

When your partner is no longer communicative, should you still be having sex? Some men whose wives lie there compliantly feel guilty about having sex if she can't verbalize her assent. In such cases, I would advise taking a close look at body language. You should be able to tell whether your partner is showing signs that he or she doesn't like what is happening, and if that happens regularly, then you should stop having sex. But just because your partner doesn't exhibit any positive signs doesn't mean that he or she isn't deriving some benefits from having sex with you; so, in such cases, I would tell you to continue. But you have to be the judge.

As Alzheimer's progresses, you, as the caregiver, will find yourself doing very personal things for your care recipient, many having to do with personal hygiene. Some people find that these activities change their perspective, and they feel less desire to have sex with the person they are caring for. This is a tricky situation because if your partner still desires sex, he or she could take your rejection very personally, so it would cause an even greater loss of self-esteem. I understand that it's not always easy to separate your loved one into two people, your life partner and this person with dementia, but to the degree that you can, do make an attempt. Perhaps, it would be helpful if while making love you kept the lights off or down low and try to use fantasy to help you become aroused. Picture the days when you were both healthy and direct your thoughts back to those times.

It's also possible that your loved one may forget what is needed for you to have sexual satisfaction. This is especially true if you are a woman who needs more than intercourse to have an orgasm. If your partner is unable to help you, you may resent the idea of having sex, as it leaves you unfulfilled. Or, if suddenly the entire responsibility of how you have sex, such as using added lubrication, falls on your shoulders, you could easily allow yourself to resent it, and thus lose the desire for sex. Such obstacles may be impossible to overcome, but at the same time, over your lifetime I'm sure you've had to overcome other such barriers. Maybe one of you broke a leg and had to wear a cast for six weeks, yet somehow you found a way to enjoy sex. Having a partner with dementia is much more complicated, I understand, but I also don't want you to give up on sex without putting up a bit of a fight. For example, even if you never used a vibrator before, perhaps this would be the time. Even if your partner is unable to use it with you, it might make having orgasms a little bit easier, and so keep you from feeling sexually frustrated.

This may also be a time to examine your sexual repertoire, for instance, the positions you use when having sex. If some become impossible, perhaps you should try others. This is true for all older couples who may find that certain positions become too difficult because of physical ailments, but it may also be true when one partner has problems with dementia.

One other problem that you might run into as a couple is that after you've had sex, the partner with dementia may forget that this has occurred and demand to have sex again. If this happens to you, you must divert your partner's attention from the desire for sex, which may not be all that strong in any case, given their age and the fact that they recently had an orgasm.

The bottom line is that the decision of when to have sex, or maybe never to have sex, is up to you. If having sex is too much of a burden, then don't. My main point is that you shouldn't abandon having sex just because your relationship has changed so dramatically. Don't assume that your sex life has to end, but instead allow yourself the freedom of choice.

If you make the decision to stop having sex, or if that decision is made for you by your spouse, don't allow this to keep you apart physically. As you'll read in this book over and over, when verbal skills disappear, touching becomes even more important. Where this can become problematic is if you don't want to have full sex any longer, but when you touch your partner, he or she thinks that is a signal to have sex. This may be confusing to both of you for a while, but if you persist at turning down advances, hopefully you'll be able to continue to touch and hug your partner without it leading to an uncomfortable situation for both of you.

While some couples continue to sleep together, some caregivers feel the need for a break, and if separate sleeping quarters are available, they will sleep apart. This is certainly understandable, but it may make your loved one feel insecure. Also, if your loved one gets up in the middle of the night or needs help, you won't be there (though a baby monitor might help with that particular situation). It is probably advisable to let your loved one's doctor know if you intend to sleep in separate rooms. If you do end up sleeping separately, one suggestion is to give your loved one a substitute, such as a stuffed animal or a pillow to hug.

In our society, older people are thought of as being sexless. When a movie features older people showing any interest in sex, it's the talk of the town, as if older people are supposed to have forgotten about sex. Yet the truth is, people can continue having sex no matter how old they are, health permitting, of course. This attitude would certainly extend to older people having sex when one partner has dementia. As I said earlier, don't allow society's attitude to have any effect on your sex life. Certainly, your relationship will change because of Alzheimer's and will continue to change. Just don't assume that Alzheimer's has to spell the end of your sex life, because then it will. Just keep an open mind and see what happens.

Masturbation

As the disease advances, as I said, some people lose all sense of inhibition. Males especially may masturbate openly. If they're doing it front of an open window or when others are around, it is not going to be acceptable. But if you're the only one witnessing this, rather than trying to always enforce a rule not to masturbate, my advice would be to walk out of the room and allow your spouse to masturbate. Yes, this is a weird situation, and you might find it quite embarrassing, but masturbation can't harm anyone, and the more sexually frustrated your spouse is, the more that frustration may show up in other ways. And, if you're tired of cleaning up after your husband, my suggestion would be to be proactive and put a towel under him rather than have a running battle and always forcing him to stop.

On the other hand, I would not recommend that you allow pornography to be part of this mix. You don't want to overstimulate your spouse, and porn does have addictive qualities. If fantasy is not enough for him, then he'll just have to deal with the situation.

If a wife asks for a vibrator, however, I would advise providing one. If a woman feels the need to have an orgasm and the only way she can do so is using the strong sensations of a vibrator, then she shouldn't have to remain sexually frustrated. I don't think this is going to be a very common request, but if it does occur, that's my opinion.

Older women also require lubrication, certainly when having intercourse, but many will need it for masturbation, as well. Here, I would definitely advise the husband of a woman with Alzheimer's to keep lubrication on hand. In fact, even if he is masturbating her, assuming she indicates that she enjoys this, he should use a lubricant to make sure that afterward she is not sore, whether or not she remembers to tell him.

JEALOUSY

When the person with Alzheimer's is put into a facility, and he or she has forgotten their spouse, an attraction for another Alzheimer's patient residing in the facility may develop. If this situation becomes mutual, it may turn into a love affair, though whether or not the two people have sex may depend on the rules of the institution. But where does that leave the spouse who is left behind? Some people are able to ignore this behavior, understanding that their spouse no longer really belongs to them. Justice Sandra Day O'Connor's son reported that his mother actually found relief in her husband's romance, as it meant that at least her husband was happy where he was. But others may feel horrible, becoming jealous or depressed.

If you run into this situation and it really bothers you, then perhaps you're going to have to curtail your visits. Yes, you feel obligated to visit, and, yes, you'll feel guilty if you don't go as often, but in the end, your mental state has to come first. Perhaps over time you'll get used to this new situation, but if your spouse no longer recognizes you and is infatuated with someone else, you're not duty bound to visit if it is going to cause you an inordinate amount of pain.

The bottom line is that when it comes to sex you have choices. There's nothing written in stone, and so if your spouse has Alzheimer's, let yourself be open to all of the possibilities. Keep in mind that as the disease progresses there are going to be changes in your sex life as a couple, so you can't really settle into a pattern. Sex is going to present one more challenge, but if you can continue your sex life together, there will also be rewards.

Your Mutual Friends

Most married people have some friends that are theirs alone and others whom they've always seen as a couple. Some of those in the former group, like the people you've maintained contact with since school days or your coworkers, may actually put more effort into reaching out to you in this time of need. Those whom you almost always saw as a couple may pull away, not because they much preferred the company of your spouse but because yours is an awkward situation. If several couples you know are going out together for dinner, do they invite only you? Are they worried that if they do extend an invitation that you might bring your spouse, who could cause them embarrassment? Are they afraid that if they're all still couples that you'll feel odd being the only "single" person there? Or, have you established a pattern of turning down such invitations, which has caused them to stop inviting you?

Having companionship is very important to a caregiver, and what I don't want to have happen to you is for any sort of misunderstanding to develop that ends up leaving you out in the cold. At this juncture in your life, it's especially important that you not be left alone, and so if it means you reaching out to them and saying please don't forget about me, then go ahead and do it. Assume that they're confused about your situation and clarify matters for them. By taking the first step, you'll be insuring that you won't be spending evenings alone for no good reason. And anytime you are asked out and can't go, for whatever reason, make sure to emphasize the fact that you want to be included in any future plans. You might even be the one to initiate a night out. That's a sure way to break the ice and avoid any confusion when it comes to your friends wondering whether or not you want to socialize with them.

When you go out with friends, politeness mandates that they ask about how you and your spouse are doing. But that may be a subject that you'd prefer to get away from for an evening. My advice would be to say a few words in answer to their question but make it clear that this evening is about you getting a break. You also shouldn't ignore the fact that you have a spouse. Don't be afraid to bring up past good times. Just remember that, for the first few times you go out with these friends, it's your job to make sure that they feel comfortable around you, so that there will never be any doubt that they invite you regularly.

I understand that these couples whom you've counted on as friends, perhaps for decades, should be the ones reaching out to you, offering you help and solace and going out of their way to remain the good friends they were in happier times. And I'm sure that some of your good friends will do that. But there are what have been called "fair-weather" friends. They enjoy socializing, but they don't want to extend a helping hand. Maybe they have a good reason, like troubles of their own. Or maybe that's just the way they are. But given that you have already lost one important friend, your spouse, my advice is not to cut these people off out of spite, not to say to yourself, "Why aren't they going the extra mile, considering all that I'm going through?" You'll get help from some people, even total strangers. But you also need companionship and some anchors to your past life, for yourself, if not for your spouse. These fair-weather friends have something to offer, and my advice is not to throw it away. They're not obligated to help you, but merely by thinking to include you in their activities they'll be offering you the opportunity for a break from your duties as caregiver.

OTHER SOCIAL CIRCLES

The two of you have interacted with other people in many ways. For example, you may have regularly attended religious services. A house of worship can offer great comfort, but if everyone stops to ask you about your spouse, that can take away from the experience. Yet you'd likely be offended if they didn't. You want you and your spouse to be in their prayers, and yet you may get so little free time away from your duties as caregiver that you don't want every experience you have outside your home to be dominated by the fact that you have a spouse with dementia.

My advice is to give a short, neutral answer like "We're coping" and quickly ask them about their lives. Try to be as upbeat as possible and try to keep the conversation flowing. You need this company, be it a book club, weekly card game, or just people you run into at the supermarket, but you need this socializing to give you a break from your role. So, to some extent it's up to you to put as positive a spin on this type of socializing as possible.

I would also suggest that you keep up with current events of all sorts, not just politics. If you want to steer a conversation away from your problems at home, you have to be equipped with the information to do so. You can't always talk about the weather. But if you know what's in the news, there will always be a topic or two you can refer to. It might be the latest movies, sports, fashion, gossip, the latest discoveries in science—you name it. As long as you're prepared, you'll be able to keep up your end of the conversation, even if you've been stuck inside the house for the last week or two.

That's not to say if you need a shoulder to cry on that you shouldn't seek out such shoulders from any group of which you're a part. If there are members of a group who sincerely want to "be there" for you, that's great. But let's say the people you play cards with once a week are really into just playing cards. They're serious card players and they don't usually discuss their problems. I suggest that you just accept such a situation, meet them to play cards, and find that shoulder to cry on elsewhere.

Maintaining Your Identity

To some extent, everyone has some difficulty maintaining a separate identity when they're part of a couple. It's easier if you're out of the house on your own a lot, for instance if you go to a job. But if you become a primary caregiver and find yourself spending most of your time at home with your spouse, the role of caregiver can become all-consuming. And, if you had any difficulties separating yourself from being Mr. and Mrs.

before an Alzheimer's diagnosis, then it's going to become even more difficult for you.

The big problem is that when you were a couple, you were clearly a separate person to your spouse. You voiced your opinions and had your own hobbies and interests. It wasn't as important to be a separate person outside of your home. I'm not saying that it isn't a good idea to have maintained activities that separated you, but it wasn't critical either. But now, with a spouse who has dementia, you must form your own identity, and preferably that identity won't be limited to that of caregiver. Let me give you one example of what I mean. Let's say you and your spouse always played tennis as a doubles team. Now, he can't play at all. Does that mean you have to stop playing the game you've enjoyed all these years? No, but it's going to take some effort on your part to make sure that doesn't happen. Either you'll have to find people who'll play singles with you or find a new partner for tennis. This example is very specific, but the truth is, you're going to have to work at setting up your own unique identity in each social circle you want to remain part of.

You Mustn't Socialize Just with Yourself

When you're talking to a spouse who doesn't understand what you're saying, it's really like talking to yourself. While there's nothing you can do about this situation, I want you to realize how important it is to make sure you don't wind up talking to yourself all day long. Everyone needs human interaction, and even though you're not actually alone, your situation is very similar to someone who is. Once you understand this new reality, you'll hopefully be better able to do something about it. But you will have to change your view of yourself as being part of a couple, because while you may still be physically joined, that may no longer be the case on other levels, such as intellectually and emotionally.

With so much on your mind, it can be easy to create a bubble around yourself. Every day, you don your role as caregiver and go about your business. But that doesn't leave room for "you." You have a void—not a physical one, of course, because actually your spouse needs more tending to than ever before. But you are faced with a void in terms of having companionship. And you need to accept the fact that you have to be proactive about filling that void. In order to be the best caregiver you can be, you need to take care of yourself physically, emotionally, and intellectually. You need to make certain that you have enough interactions with other people to recharge your batteries. If you need someone to talk to about your situation, or about the news, or if you need a shoulder to cry on, seek out other people. Make sure that you maintain communication with the outside world so that your situation doesn't become overwhelming.

For the LGBT Community

As I write this, more and more states are legalizing gay marriage, but nevertheless, most gay couples are not married. However, the emotional attachment you have for each other is not affected by your marital status, and the difficulties you have with Alzheimer's may be more acute for several reasons.

For example, if a gay person has not come out, the pressures of a serious disease like Alzheimer's may make his or her life more problematic. There is a host of issues that are going to have to be addressed, such as doctor visits, hospital visiting rights, and a whole array of financial matters, and sometimes the only way to get around them will be to acknowledge the relationship. Many of these issues will also affect openly gay couples, as most hospitals will not release medical information to an unmarried partner. Keep in mind that even without being married, there are papers that can be signed, like a power of attorney, which will help you get through such situations. But such papers can only be signed either before dementia strikes or in the early stages. If you wait too long, no attorney will be able to certify that your partner was of sound mind and therefore legally able to sign such documents.

Many gay men and women do not have a committed partner, and finding a caregiver can be very difficult. They may not have children, and some have become estranged from other relatives because of their sexual identity, so that even though they are in dire need of assistance, relatives one might expect to be of help refuse. And while any single individual is going to encounter more stress in caring for a sick parent, more gays are single and so more likely to run into this set of problems. Additionally, the sexual issues that I wrote about between husbands and wives could be further complicated if the relationship has never been legally sanctified.

Research has shown that many gays who were reluctant to come out of the closet will return to the closet once they hit a certain age. Since it was never easy for them to be openly gay, and as they gain more responsibilities in their work life, they may decide it's easier not to be open about their sexuality. This solves some problems when it comes to discrimination when rising up the ranks, but it creates others when it comes to health matters, as a partner cannot be fully included in the process. The best time to address this type of situation is before you run into any health problems.

In other words, being a solo caregiver or obtaining caregiving for oneself, which is already very difficult for anyone, may end up being even more difficult for gays and lesbians. My advice to you is to reach out for as much support as you can in order to address and accommodate these extra burdens. I never tell gays and lesbians who come to see me that they must come out. On the other hand, if a gay or lesbian caregiver is really in need of assistance dealing with Alzheimer's, the gay community might offer a potential support network whose benefits should not be ignored.

All caregivers are under tremendous stress. If you end up being under even more stress because of discrimination, family dynamics, or potential isolation, at the very least you have to recognize the source of that added stress and take steps to alleviate it in whichever ways make the most sense to you.

5

When You're Taking Care of a Parent or Other Relative

You owe your parents a lot. They created you, took care of you, and made countless sacrifices for you. Now the tables are turned because one of them has been stricken with Alzheimer's. Aside from the added burdens in terms of time, energy, and finances, there is certainly a psychological cost. You've probably always looked at this parent for psychological support. It started when you ran to Mom or Dad when you skinned your knee, but even as an adult, you still looked to them for reassurance on a range of issues. Now that parent's support has been pulled out from under you, and instead the role of parent has been thrust upon you as you take charge of their care. Unquestionably, this adds to the difficulty of your situation. (At this point I must recognize that not every parent/ child relationship is perfect. If you and your parent with Alzheimer's have had a contentious relationship, that unfortunate fact is going to create an entirely different set of circumstances if the responsibility of taking care of them suddenly falls on your shoulders. I would strongly advise anyone in such a situation to obtain professional counseling. While counseling may not be able to change the entire underlying relationship, it will certainly help you feel less conflicted about your duties as caregiver.)

Children who must suddenly take on the role of parent must seek a middle ground. No matter their mental state, your parents are still your parents. Thus, you can't distance yourself from the patient you are caring for the way a professional can. Your emotions are going to play an important role. If your mom is screaming at you, perhaps the way she did when you were a child, perhaps even using the same hurtful phrases like "You're so fat" that used to cause you so much pain, you are going to react emotionally, at least while you first begin to adapt to the role of caregiver. After so many years of being programmed that way, it's just not possible to shut down your emotional triggers. That's not to say that you can't find ways of coping with such situations, but first you have to recognize what is happening, and then you have to work at changing your reactions.

Of course, your history with your parents will make caregiving much more difficult in myriad different ways. To see your father crying, for example, will be very hard on you, because to you your father was a bulwark of strength. To have to change a parent's soiled clothes is going to be much tougher than if you were caring for a stranger or even a spouse. To have to hand-feed a parent or simply to have to watch your mother or father staring into space when you clearly remember when they were so full of life will be very trying for you.

Since this situation can continue for years, you're going to have to steel yourself against these emotions. But at the same time, you don't want to harden your heart to the point where you forget all that this person means to you. This is going to require you to live in the past and the present at the same time. Try to rely on your memories to lift your spirits, and, at the same time, remove the focus of your emotions from the present.

Easier said than done, you say? Of course that's true, and that is why you can't do this successfully without preparing yourself.

Have you ever been to a wake where there are lots of poster boards filled with pictures of the deceased that were taken at various memorable times, like at birthday parties or family get-togethers? (Some funeral homes these days even have the technical equipment in place to show videos.) What happens is that all the family members look at those pictures and share those positive memories, and it makes grieving a little easier. I'm going to suggest that you do something similar, but you might need some help doing it. These days people love DVDs, but DVDs need special equipment to watch, and that requires more time. What I would suggest is that you make a book about your parent that would include pictures as well as written memories of your mother or father provided by various family members. See if you can put this book in chronological order and keep it in a place where you can easily reach it. Then, once or twice a day, take it out and look at a page. Try to immerse yourself in one particular day, be it a special one or an average day that for some reason stands out, and keep flooding your brain with positive memories. Use those memories to help balance out the scenes that may be playing themselves out in front of you.

Bear in mind that if you're having a bad time with your parent, for whatever reason, and you're not prepared with these memory aids, it's going to be very difficult to use the past to put a more pleasant glow on the present. But if you do what I'm suggesting, and also add a little willpower, you will be able to change the negative emotions you feel.

Let me repeat that I'm a behavioral therapist. I'm not just saying these things—I know they work. Just as I know they won't be of any use unless you make the proper preparations. Depending on when you're reading this book, maybe you can start your emotional preparation while your parent still has lucid moments and when he or she can clearly remember the past. Alzheimer's tends to attack current memories more than older ones, so you might even have some limited success asking questions of a parent who's had Alzheimer's for some time. When you bring up the past, try to use a voice recorder or camera to record what they are saying at the time and try to get down as many details as you can about the parent's memories of family vacations, parties, and other highlights. If you can get their voice or image recorded when talking about these events, you can play these back later on.

It may be tempting to think that somehow Alzheimer's will stop its course and your parent will always be able to keep some semblance of their old selves. It might happen, but the odds are that it won't, so rather than bury your head in the sand, ostrich-like, be realistic and salvage as much of your parent's memories as you can, starting the moment you receive that dreaded diagnosis.

GRANDCHILDREN

Of course, there's another reason to do this, and that's if you have children or intend to have them. Depending on their ages, you want to make sure they remember your parent in the best possible light. It's going to be hard explaining to them what is going on with Grandma or Grandpa. I wouldn't advise concentrating on the present. In fact, I would say it's more important, for their sake, to talk about the good times of the past.

It's time for a little aside here about the importance of talking about the past. For most of mankind's time on this planet, our history has been kept alive not through history books, but through an oral tradition. Our brains are very well equipped to remember stories if we hear them enough times. You can do a better job of making moments of your past, and your parent's past, come alive by speaking about them. Children like to be told stories, especially when these stories are about people they know. They don't have to be full of drama, like a television show or movie. They can be simple stories, but if they're repeated often enough, they will become a part of the children's lives, too.

This type of storytelling is something that we should be doing throughout our lives, but often we're pressed for time or just don't think of it. Now that you have a strong incentive, I suggest you put more effort into this process. Make it a family affair. Bring in your siblings, aunts and uncles, even next-door neighbors—anyone who has a story to tell about your family should be made a part of the oral history. And, if possible, give these stories a permanent life by actually recording them.

In my book, *Musically Speaking: A Life Through Song*, I use the music that played a role in my life to weave my biography. At the end of the book, I suggested that readers make a CD of the important music that figured in the various stages of their life. Obviously, to do something like this with the music of your parent's life would not only be meaningful to you, and would help your children to gain a better understanding of their grandparents, but it would also be something that might be enjoyable to your parent. These would be songs that might evoke memories for them, and anything that might prompt their brain to recall something pleasant from the past is worth pursuing. While Alzheimer's damages the brain's pathways that are required to use words, that might not be true for other types of memories that music could trigger.

Several of the people I know who are current caregivers told me that they sing old-time songs to their parent. It has a very soothing influence on them, much like the way you croon to a baby to get them to sleep. Even if your parent can't tell you that they remember the music you are singing or playing on a CD, there's a good chance that it is getting though and having a positive effect.

Your Siblings

In most situations, one sibling takes care of the parent with Alzheimer's. That may be the case because he or she has the most room, or the deepest pockets, or because that sibling still lives in the parental home. It would be great if all the siblings shared equally in the care of their parent, but that's just not always possible for reasons of geography, marital status, children, or employment. It may also be better for someone whose memory is failing to stay in the place where they are the most comfortable, best know their way around, and perhaps where the home has been best prepared for them, in terms of safety.

If one sibling becomes the main caregiver, the others should kick in as much as possible. But, of course, sometimes that doesn't occur, and resentment builds up and it can easily turn into a big problem. How to handle family squabbles is a subject worthy of an entire book, because there are too many permutations of who did or said what when. But there are some general issues that may arise that I want to cover.

The first issue could be labeled "martyrdom." The sibling who has full-time care of the parent tells other family members that everything is under control and no help is needed. That, of course, is not true, because taking care of someone with Alzheimer's is tough, and help is most certainly needed.

There could be many reasons for turning down sibling help. It could be an issue of control. The person in whose home the parent resides prefers for everything to be done in a certain way, and rather than risk having the sugar bowl not put back in its place, he or she would prefer to do it all. Such an attitude lets the other siblings off the hook. The easiest thing for them to do is to give in and see this parent only occasionally. It might be the easiest solution, but it's not the most ethical, nor the most beneficial to all parties concerned. It doesn't matter how obstinate this sibling caretaker is, he or she does need help. Maybe this person is putting up all these false barriers because of a fear that help won't really be forthcoming, so they steel themselves against the possibility of being disappointed. Maybe each sibling has settled into certain roles, perhaps brought about by birth order, so that the older sister, for example, has always shouldered more of the burdens and expects it to remain this way.

Let's get down to the heart of the problem. Perhaps this oldest sister always hosted Thanksgiving, for whatever reason, and it was a bit unfair, but in the end, it really isn't that big a deal. Taking care of a parent with Alzheimer's is a big deal. Help is needed, and the siblings must be forceful in providing that assistance. This can be an overwhelming task, and even if Mom is going to remain at this sister's house, the other siblings must make a real effort to shoulder some of this burden.

The best way to handle such situations is by a family meeting. Try to iron out all the wrinkles so that the responsibility of caring for a parent is shared as much as possible. You must all be realistic, however, because there is never going to be a way to share this task exactly. You must accept as a given that one sibling is going to end up doing more. But if you all talk about it, if you all acknowledge the situation, and if you are clearly doing as much as you can, hard feelings can be avoided.

If it seems that the level of conflict is too high for you to settle this among yourselves, I would suggest calling in an arbitrator: an aunt or uncle who is respected by everyone, or maybe a cousin who is a lawyer. Or, perhaps if there is one, you can use the family lawyer as a non-partial arbitrator. Whatever you do, don't let bad feelings fester. At some point, the rift could become so great that it may never be healed, and that's the last thing your ailing parent would want to happen.

For family members who live far away, the care of their parent is going to have an unreal quality to it. They won't see how difficult it is to handle the day-in day-out care. And, if they haven't seen their parent in a while, they may not be aware how much deterioration has taken place in the interim. Such family members also end up contributing the least, and not necessarily because of bad faith, but just because of the geographic limitations. Because of this, I'm going to make a suggestion that isn't going to be easy, and that suggestion is that they give up their vacations in order to fill in as caretakers.

We need to examine the psychology caused by distance to fully understand this. If you don't live with an Alzheimer's patient every day, you can't possibly understand or fully appreciate what an undertaking this really is. If you work hard fifty weeks of the year, to give up the freedom offered by a vacation will be a major sacrifice, especially to your nuclear family. While it's true that for your sister who changes your mother's diaper several times a day this task has become easier just because it's become part of her routine, it's something that you need to take the responsibility of doing, if not to help, at least so that you fully appreciate what your sister is going through.

A Word about Advice

Actually, this section is not a word of advice, but some words about *giving* advice, as well as taking it. The person who is the main caregiver, call her Sally, obviously knows the most about Mom's condition. It is going to be a little hard for Sally to accept advice. Let's say Sally's brother, Bob, has done some research on the Web and says that the best way to handle Mom is by doing such and such. But Sally is going to feel that she knows what is best because it's part of her everyday routine. Now, Bob is only trying to be helpful, and he wants to alleviate any guilt he feels by at least contributing some advice. But this can turn into a vicious cycle where the caregiver feels put upon rather than helped, rightly or wrongly I might add.

The point I'm trying to make is to be very gentle when giving advice. As helpful as you might want to be, if you're not taking full responsibility for the care of your parent, then you have to allow the caregiver some leeway. If you feel that the caregiver is making a mistake, I would go back to my suggestion of finding a family arbitrator, like an aunt or uncle. Whatever you do—and by "you" I mean the caregiver and any other relatives—don't turn this into a fight. Don't allow your ego to get in the way, and try to see all sides.

Sibling Rivalry

In some families, the siblings vie for their parent's attention, and that causes what is known as sibling rivalry. To the extent that such forces make each sibling strive to outdo the other and each becomes better at whatever it is they do, sibling rivalry can be a positive force. But it can also become exaggerated and cause much unnecessary friction. Of course, if the effects of sibling rivalry have been at play since all the siblings were young, it's going to be impossible to just shut down this source of conflict. But having a parent who has Alzheimer's, the family is faced with a very real and very serious issue, and so everyone must try his or her hardest to work together and stop competing against one another.

The bottom line should be what is best for Mom or Dad, although what is best might not always be obvious. You might be in a situation where several options all offer different advantages. If you can't settle these differences peacefully among yourselves, then again, I say bring in a mediator. This is a situation where there are plenty of contributions everybody can make, and the last thing that you need is to start a fight that will make caregiving less efficient.

Be aware that certain patterns of behavior that arose when you were much younger may still be at play, even if you are not fully aware of them. Sibling rivalry can be very strong and obvious to all, or it can be mild and remain an undercurrent that has caused some conflict but nothing really major. However, when you are under stress—and having to watch one of your parents succumb to the ravages of this disease is certainly stressful— a slight crack in the relationships among siblings can grow. Small squabbles can become full-scale fights. What you all must do is take a step back and recognize the underlying cause of these conflicts. Even if it's not apparent, assume that there is some underlying cause, and don't get on your high horse. As I've been saying, if the siblings can't do this on their own, if the squabbles are getting out of hand, it is time to get someone else to step in and act as peacemaker.

OTHER FAMILY MEMBERS

I've suggested using other family members to mediate disputes, but, of course, your parent may have a brother or sister who ends up being a troublemaker. There's that old saying about too many cooks spoiling the soup, and if everyone has an opinion, it can drive you, as the main caregiver, a bit crazy. All this advice you're getting may be well-intentioned, but if the source is the fear that aunts and uncles may have about their own mortality, then it may be counterproductive.

In situations where an older relative tries to pull seniority, I would go back to advice I've given elsewhere in this book, which is to use your parent's doctor as your ally. If the doctor who is in charge of the patient's care endorses the care you are giving, then everyone else has to leave you alone. Here again, don't start a fight with these relatives. Try to deflect their attention, not only because they are relatives and so do have some claim on your parent, but also because they might be able to provide you with some real assistance. This will only be possible if you're all on good terms.

OTHER RELATIONSHIPS

Most caregivers are part of the immediate family, but certainly not all. In fact, I have a good friend who never had children, and it's his niece and nephew who live not too far away who make the constant trips in to see him and take him to the doctor. They are not with him all the time, but they're very involved. You expect to take care of a spouse or parent, but if your relationship is a little more distant, what are your responsibilities? How guilty should you feel when you can't be with your relative all the time? Do you turn your life upside down or just do whatever you can?

Obviously, there's no one answer to these questions because the circumstances can be so varied. But no matter your relationship, and that includes just being a good friend, you can only do what you can do, and if you're contributing to this person's well-being, you mustn't feel guilty that you can't take on the responsibility for being a full-time caregiver. The caregiving you are providing is a blessing for your relative and the other caregivers in his or her life, but when you reach your limit, you have to pull back.

Consider all this in the light of the opposite reaction. There are many people who won't get involved in caretaking at all just so that they don't become pulled in too deeply. By staying away from the situation completely, they don't risk having to do more than they can. But, of course, by doing little to nothing at all, they are placing a burden on other relatives and friends, or the government. The person doing whatever he or she can is contributing both to this person and to society. So when you reach your limit and have to pull back, it's okay. At least you did something; you put in effort and time and money, and so you deserve nothing but credit.

When Your Parent Lives Far Away

Some parents choose to live in other places than their children, like those who move to warmer climes after they retire. Others stay put while their children move away. Any distance can add to the overall stress of taking care of aging parents, but if that distance is far enough to require a plane ride, possibly even one to another country or continent, that adds all sorts of complications to the responsibility of caregiving.

If you find yourself in such a situation, the first thing you must do is be proactive, hopefully before your parents' health declines. You need to create a network of eyes, ears, and hands in the community where your parents reside that you trust and can count on. For example, your parents will probably have a physician, but is he or she the best one? On one of your visits, see that your parents have a doctor's appointment scheduled for that time period so that you can accompany them, both to make your own assessment and to make a personal connection. If you have any legal paperwork the doctor might need to see, like a health proxy, it would be better to show it to the doctor in person so as to make sure that this doctor will communicate directly with you by phone if something were to happen. Just because this sort of paperwork is supposed to work doesn't mean it will. But if you've established a personal rapport with the doctor, and shown him or her the paperwork ahead of time, then all should be fine.

It would also be a good idea to check out support options like in-home food delivery (meals-on-wheels or whatever the local alternative is) and in-home services such as bathing, physical therapy, or cleaning. You might want to visit local assisted-care facilities, especially if both of your parents live some distance away from you. (If something were to happen to a single parent's health that required institutionalization, you might relocate him or her to a facility near you, though that would assume they were sufficiently healthy to be transported.) You might also want to find a lawyer in your parents' area to whom you could give a power of attorney and who could then act as a surrogate for you in case you couldn't get to your parents in a timely manner.

I have a German friend who lives in the United States, whose parents remained in Germany. As they became older and had more health problems, he found that a local pastor, a connection he had made on behalf of his parents, ended up playing a crucial role. He provided the link to many services, was able to give comfort, and even searched the apartment when certain papers were needed. That's not to say that you will always find someone like this, but it's certainly true that you will never find this help if you don't look for it.

The Fear Factor

By now, nearly everyone is aware that genetics play a large role in your health. If a parent comes down with any disease, the odds that the children will inherit the same trait, and hence be more likely to suffer the same fate, grow much higher. This possibility could translate into a mere apprehension or grow exponentially into an overpowering fear. When that happens, the children of parents with a serious disease like Alzheimer's may become paralyzed. Rather than the family coming together, some or all of the siblings try to hide from the situation. I know of situations where this had occurred.

As I've said before, fear is an emotion that can be difficult to overcome because it can cause paralysis. Of course, you have to recognize what is occurring in order to do anything about it. If one sibling is avoiding the situation, it's easy to think it's due to laziness or selfishness and not fear. The best thing to do in such a situation is for the person who is afraid to speak up. The end result may be that he or she is forced to face up to their fear, but as the saying goes, the brave man only dies once, while the coward dies a thousand deaths, so it's always better to face one's fears.

Since it might not be possible to know how much fear each of the siblings is facing, I'd suggest that you hold a family conference and discuss this subject. There's no doubt that each sibling will be somewhat fearful, and admitting this fact might help any who are paralyzed by their fear to open up. Maybe such siblings could be convinced to go for therapy. Or maybe they could be lured into devoting more time to caregiving if more shared support were available during the first few visits.

FAMILIES ARE IMPORTANT

I want to end by saying that when a family member is diagnosed with Alzheimer's, or any serious illness, this should be a time when everybody pulls together. It's sad when the opposite happens, and you must work to see that it doesn't. Family dynamics are complicated, any number of triggers can set off arguments, and the stress of Alzheimer's can put all or some family members on a hair trigger so that it doesn't take much to cause an explosion. Everyone needs to try their hardest to make sure this doesn't happen. It's bad enough that Alzheimer's has to claim one family member, but it would be terrible if it also managed to split a family apart entirely.

6

Dealing with Professional Caregivers

When I was a young child, ten to be exact, I lost control over my life. I was sent to Switzerland to escape the Nazis and lost my entire family. As an orphan living in a school, I really had no say over much of anything. I had to be grateful that strangers were keeping me safe and fed and that I had a roof over my head, so the idea of being a rebellious teenager just never entered my mind. But when you've gone through a period like that, when you finally do gain back control over your life, you tend to hold onto it. I say this to let you know that I fully understand how hard it can be to give up control. And that's especially true when it involves someone you love who needs all the tender loving care possible.

GETTING HELP EARLY

At the same time, having a loved one with Alzheimer's is going to mean giving up some control. You might think that you can do it all, but you can't. You're going to need all the help you can get, and my advice is the sooner you start reaching out to others, the better. The reason I say this is that having outsiders come into your home is a challenge. You have to learn how to handle this situation and how to make sure that your care recipient is getting the best care. The more advanced the disease, the less able you will be to control the situation. If help arrives when you're overwhelmed, you're likely to just hand over control because you physically and mentally can't take it any more. But if you bring in outside help at an earlier stage, you can integrate this help into your everyday routine. You can find people who will do the best job. You can be "professional" about it. So rather than fight this milestone, rather than say to yourself, "As long as I can handle everything, I'll feel as close to normal as possible," I'm advising you to do the reverse. Normalcy isn't in the cards for you any longer, so trying to hold on to it is counterproductive. The sooner you start to adapt to your new non-normal situation, the better.

Caring for someone with Alzheimer's is going to sap your reserves of strength and sanity. I don't care how strong you are, there is no getting around this fact. So rather than risk burnout, begin integrating help as soon as possible. Test the waters. Try out different agencies. Join support groups and try to learn as much as you can about the help available in your area. If there's a fund-raiser for Alzheimer's research, attend and meet as many people as you can. Start building your network of sources of help right at the beginning, while you still have the time and the energy.

For example, you may meet someone who has a great in-home care-taker, but the patient has deteriorated so much that he or she is going to a care facility in the near future. Well, in that case, you make sure that this great caretaker is going to come to you next. That may mean that you have to hire this person a few months before you'd planned on doing so. But if that means you'll get a great caregiver without doing a ton of research and spending hours interviewing people who are wrong for the job, and maybe out of desperation having to settle for someone who is second best, then that will be money well spent.

Or maybe you'll find someone who has a good caretaker but doesn't need or can't afford to keep this caretaker full time. Since the caretaker needs full-time work, there's a chance that this person will go elsewhere. Perhaps by offering to split this person between the two of you, there'll be the equivalent of a full-time job and you can both use her services. Or there might be someone who has full-time help who wouldn't mind taking care of two people for short periods so that you could drop off your care recipient (and pay for the care during that time period, of course) to give yourself a couple of hours a week to do some shopping. So even if you don't hire anyone, at least nose around and be open to testing the waters. You never know what you may find.

How the Patient Feels

One obstacle you might encounter may come from the Alzheimer's patient himself. He or she may not want some stranger to be involved in his or her life. Particularly, in the early stages, when the patient is in full control of their faculties much of the time, they're quite likely not going to want a stranger around. They're going to want to maintain their independence They won't want to admit that control over their life is sliding away from them. Such an attitude is fully understandable, and your tendency is going to be to give in, especially if you share this same reluctance. But as we all learned from an Aesop's fable, the time to stock the pantry is in summer when the food is available, not once winter comes and there's nothing left to harvest. If you are harried because you can't cope with your spouse or parent, how easy is it going to be to find help? At that point, you'll be more likely to make a poor choice. But if you start early enough, even if you do make a mistake, you'll have time to rectify it.

So just because the person in your care may object to the presence of an outside caregiver, don't let this be reason enough to stop you. You don't want to paint too grim a picture of the future for your loved one, that's understandable, but you have a duty to be realistic. And you know what is likely to happen? The patient who objected so vigorously is going to appreciate the help and not having to bother you with every little thing. People are adverse to change, but given some time to adapt, they'll understand that change can be a good thing.

NO TIMETABLE

It can be hard to come to grips with the fact that with Alzheimer's there is no going back or even standing still for very long. There's no exact timetable either. The person you are caring for could remain stable for some time, or a month from now he or she could be in very bad shape. There's no road map to follow, so my advice is to make as much progress as you can in terms of getting help while there's still some daylight left.

You also have to realize that the person with Alzheimer's is not alone on this journey. It's not all about the patient; it involves the entire family and especially you as the main caregiver. You're going to be making plenty of sacrifices, so don't feel the least bit guilty about doing something for yourself, like setting up some assistance. You have to marshal your forces for this long journey. If you don't protect your strength, you'll never make it.

You also have to think of your own health. If your physical condition is weakened, you could develop a serious health problem of your own. This is actually very common among caregivers who tend to neglect their own health. Not only would that be terrible for your sake, this could have a very negative impact on the person you're caring for. Your mom might have to be sent to a facility long before she otherwise might have been if you're no longer able to care for her.

I'm not trying to paint an overly bleak picture here. I just know that it is part of human nature to put certain things off, particularly if they're not all that pleasant and require spending what may be scarce financial resources. However, given the circumstances of Alzheimer's, it is essential that you overcome your natural reticence and allow yourself to be proactive.

Adjusting

Now we come to the meat and potatoes of this chapter, adjusting to having a caregiver in your home. Of course, if you have the right person, it won't be difficult at all. If you have someone who is experienced in caring for people with Alzheimer's and who is pleasant to be around, any time you have spent worrying about getting a reliable caregiver will have been for nothing. If that's what has transpired in your situation, perhaps you can skip reading the rest of this chapter. But, let's face it, this sort of match rarely goes completely smoothly. If 50 percent of all marriages end in divorce—relationships that started off as loving—it's far from certain that your relationship with this outside person is going to be flawless. On the other hand, you are not marrying this person, so set your sights a little lower. As long as they do offer you help, and as long as it seems the person you're caring for is doing okay under their charge, that's all you really need to expect. If you get more, great, but if you get that minimum, you need to be more accepting. In all probability, this person is not making very much money. (That's especially true if you hired the caregiver through an agency, which is getting a large cut.) You can't expect that person to give exactly the type of care you would give because they don't have a personal connection to the person whom they are tending.

By the way, in case you think that I don't understand the mentality of someone in this position, I need to inform you that while I was in the orphanage in Switzerland, I earned a diploma in Swiss housekeeping. When I first came to this country, I worked as a housekeeper for seventy-five cents an hour to support myself and my young daughter. As it happened, I remained friends with the couple that first employed me, as I was very grateful to them. But I know what it is like to be a domestic worker, though I also know that cleaning floors is a lot less psychologically tiring than taking care of someone with Alzheimer's. And that's something you should appreciate as well.

THE ART OF DIPLOMACY

Your number-one goal with regards to the "outsider" in whom you are trusting the care of your loved one is for your loved one to feel comfortable with and comforted by this person. If you are too demanding or too picky, you will have a difficult time feeling confident when you're out of the house that this goal is being met. You probably won't be able to trust what your care recipient says, because he or she might have some difficulty telling what is real and what is not. Your husband might complain bitterly about a caregiver who is perfect in your eyes but is seen as an enemy by your spouse because of her need to keep your loved one from doing things that might cause himself harm. On the other hand, if your loved one can't remember whether or not he or she was ever served lunch, there's no way for you to know besides trusting the person you hired.

Of course, these days it is possible to place secret video cameras so that you can see what is taking place, to be viewed either live or recorded for later viewing. My instinct is to tell you not to do that. Frankly, this comes in part from me not being very technically savvy, so I'd be afraid of all the necessary equipment. But I also believe that installing this type of surveillance is indicative of mistrust, which is not a good way to begin such a relationship or to make it work. On the other hand, I have to admit that if it gives you peace of mind, and especially if you've had some bad experiences, it's something to consider.

I would say that having hidden cameras around would be more appropriate if your care recipient has developed a tendency to be mean or act out in inappropriate ways. Such behavior is going to tax the patience of any caregiver. You yourself might be very upset by it from time to time. So, it could be a good idea to make sure that the person you've hired is handling such behavior in an appropriate manner. Now, that manner doesn't have to be exactly the way you would do it, it just can't be in a way that puts your loved one in harm's way.

Here's another personal story that I want to pass on because it shows my philosophy of life. My daughter was getting married. The most famous shop to buy a wedding dress was, at the time, located in Brooklyn, near where my coauthor Pierre lives. After looking at the dresses, we stopped by his house. I had hired a car and driver for the afternoon. When we got to Pierre's, I invited the driver in to join us for coffee and cake. Later, my daughter asked Pierre whether this was a driver I had used many times. The answer was that I'd never used him before and there was every chance I would never have him drive me again. So why did I not leave him sitting outside in the car? Why do I always make sure that a driver is not going to go hungry if I'm being taken somewhere for a meal, to the point where I will often bring a banana to give the driver just in case he can't leave his car and get a bite?

It goes back to what I just told you, as a result of my having been a domestic worker. My status may have changed tremendously from those days, but I'm the same person. I certainly wanted to be treated like a person back in those days, and so I never forget to treat everyone around me as if they are complete equals. If a friend had been driving me to Brooklyn, I most certainly would have asked him in, so why not the driver I didn't know?

What do I get in return for following the golden rule? I can always rely on the people I work with because they never feel as if I'm cheating them. Of course, there are people who don't care how they're treated. They have a chip on their shoulder or some other psychological problem, and no matter how nice you are, you are going to regret having had them in your employ, or as neighbors, or sitting next to you on the bus. There are people who will sometimes take advantage of other people, which is why you might choose to install video cameras. On the other hand, the likelihood of needing a security camera is pretty small, and if you treat people well, you'll usually be afforded the same respect.

Another piece of advice I would give is when you're interviewing caregivers, make sure that you don't do all the talking. If you have instructions or want to tell this person all about your mother, you can do that at some later time after you've made the decision to engage them. But in an interview, you want to learn as much about the person you're hiring as you can. The only way to do that is to ask them questions and then—this is the important part—listen carefully to the responses you are given. You can learn a lot about a person that way, but if you're too wrapped up in what you want to say, you'll miss both information and vital clues. Keep in mind that a job interview is not a social call where you get to tell this person about all the time and effort you've put into taking care of your loved one. The only goal is to try to ascertain whether or not the person in front of you can do a capable job of assisting you in this crucial task.

I would suggest that you write down a set of questions ahead of time so that you remember the important ones. You want to know about their past experience working with people with dementia. You'll want to ask them if they ever had any incidents with someone in their care. You want to know that if the person they are caring for gets abusive, how they approach and handle such situations. Try to come up with questions that don't allow for yes or no answers. Try to make the person speak in full sentences so that you really get a picture of them. You can write out little scenarios, such as "If my mom refused to eat lunch, how would you handle it?" By carefully evaluating their response and observing both their verbal and nonverbal signals, you'll learn a lot about them.

On the other hand, don't worry too much about their background. It's likely that this person doesn't share your background. Their lifestyle may be very different from yours. But that doesn't have very much to do with whether or not they would make a good caregiver.

When you check their references (and always check, because what good are references if you don't call those previous employers?), you want to obtain the same type of information as in the interview. Unexpected incidents are almost bound to come up with someone with Alzheimer's, and there's no one perfect way to handle these various types of incidents. But you want to have confidence that this person expects them and won't fly off the handle in reaction to something your care recipient does or says.

Sometimes you just have to be practical. Let's say your father has taken to saying things that are racist, even though he never did so before dementia hit him. If that's the case, you are going to have to find someone of his race to take care of him because no matter how thick someone says their skin is, if they are being verbally abused on a daily basis, it's going to take a toll, and in the long run, they're not going to be able to give your loved one the proper care. Or, if your father is always making passes at women you hire, then you should seek out a man to take care of him. Occasional inappropriate behavior can be handled, but if it's constant, it's going to wear down the patience of anyone who is not a family member (and, of course, even a loving family member's patience will occasionally wear thin).

If and when you find the perfect (or near-perfect) caregiver, treat this person well. Even if you can't afford to give them a raise, make sure to bring home little presents, ask them about their family, and do everything in your power to make them feel like they are one of the family, so that they won't leave you just because someone else offers them a few dollars more per hour. Of course, you may not be able to prevent that from happening, but the better you treat them from the beginning, the more insurance against them leaving you are purchasing with your kind gestures. (And, if you're not paying a "gem" very much money, don't advertise to the world how good she is; otherwise, you'll be advertising to someone else that they should outbid you for her services.)

You also need to be careful about the job description when you first hire someone. Is this person going to be responsible only for the care of the person with Alzheimer's, or are other more general housekeeping duties part of the job? Give it some thought. Finding someone to help you clean is likely to be far easier than finding a person capable of handing someone with Alzheimer's. Whatever you do, don't hire someone intending to ask them to help with other chores without being very up front about it; otherwise, conflicts are sure to arise.

You may also have to be protective with regards to this employee vis-a-vis your other relatives. If this person's job is only to take care of your mother, say, and your sister comes to visit and starts giving her orders that are not part of the job description, that could cause a serious conflict. So, make sure other relatives understand exactly what this person is supposed to be doing so that no misunderstandings arise.

KEEPING YOUR DISTANCE

I've been telling you that it's good if this caregiver becomes part of the family, and I do agree with that, but be careful about getting too close, too early. You may discover after a month that this person is just not right for the job. Maybe she starts to come late every other day. Or she spends too much time talking on her cell phone. If you've gotten too close too fast, you're going to have a harder time either exerting control or getting rid of her. So, in the early stages of her employment, maintain your status of being the boss. If this person turns out to be someone worthy of being considered a "member of the family," you can always make relationship changes later on. And that status will be more appreciated if it's earned than if it's granted too soon.

In your role as employer, be specific when it comes to instructions. You should definitely have a written list for emergencies—who to call and what to do—but it's a good idea to write out any other instructions you might have, such as what foods can and cannot be served, when medications are to be given, and so forth. Also, you might want to leave daily written instructions as well, such as when to bathe the patient, though these may eventually be communicated orally once you have full confidence that this person listens to what you tell them. Leave any such lists where they're easily accessible, not stuffed in a drawer, but out in the open.

There are several advantages to giving the person such a list. First, it will permit you to make sure that you've given all the proper instructions. Also, it will help the person you hired not to forget those instructions. A written list is also a "witness" in case of disagreements. This person can't say to you, "You never told me to do this or that" if there's a written list to prove otherwise.

INITIALLY DON'T BE A SOFTIE

Once you have an employee, you become a "boss." You don't want to act too bossy, but you also don't want to appear to be a softie because that will encourage this employee to take advantage of you. I'm not saying every employee would, but some might. If you set the stage early on, and if this person knows that you mean business, then those early limits you set should hold. However, if you are always giving in or giving mixed signals, particularly right from the beginning, it will be very hard to regain control. Thus, while you're getting to know each other, make sure to don yourself with the robes of authority. Hopefully, this is a role that you won't have to maintain, but being fully in charge initially will be helpful to everybody. Your employee will be less likely to find herself in a situation where the job is going to be taken away from her, and you'll be less likely to have to go through the process of finding someone to replace her.

Of course, as every parent who employs a nanny or baby sitter to look after their child knows all too well, no matter how good the person you've hired is, there will be times when he or she will notify you at the last minute that they can't come to work. Emergencies happen, so you have to be prepared with a back-up plan. If you prepare for such situations, not only will they not be as traumatic, but they'll happen less often. That's just the way fate seems to roll the dice, because if you're unprepared, foul-ups tend to happen more often than not.

The Drop-In Caregiver

Up to now, I've addressed the issue of a regular-care assistant, but in all likelihood you may also encounter people who come into your home from time to time, such as a physical therapist, a nurse who administers medication, or a social worker. Such visits are a bit like a doctor's visit. If you've been encountering problems of any sort, you'll want to write down your questions so that when this person is with you, you can get the answers you need. If you think of your questions after this person has left, it doesn't do you much good.

On the other hand, such specialists have limited time to spend with you, so you don't want to flood them with questions or complaints that have nothing to do with why they are there. That's another reason to have a written list of items to discuss, so that you can make sure you're raising only appropriate issues.

You and the Staff at a Facility

If your loved one is in a facility, you'll come into contact with the caregivers there on a regular basis. As with a hired home caregiver, it's equally, if not more important, to maintain good relations with facility caregivers and staff members. The reason it could be more important is that most of the time you won't be on the facility grounds to supervise. Also, if your loved one is in a facility, he or she probably doesn't have much ability to speak up for him or herself. Finally, someone in the final stages of Alzheimer's may have some personality disorders that may make them harder to deal with. The people in the facility are of course professionals who do this every day, but it's not an easy job, and the people who are most closely involved with your loved one—in other words not the medical staff but the aides—are probably not paid very much.

In such situations, you have a dual role. One part of your role is to ascertain that your care recipient is getting the proper care and attention. That means you're going to have to ask questions and be a bit nosy, which is not always going to make you all that popular. However, since your care recipient won't be able to communicate very well, if at all, you have to be his or her personal ambassador toward the staff. You have to make the staff see this patient through the lens of the family members who come to visit. So, the nicer and more diplomatic you are, the more little gifts you bring, the more polite you are toward them, the better treatment your loved one is likely to get. It doesn't matter whether Medicaid, a private insurance company, or your bank account is paying, what you can offer when you're there is another type of currency that can have a lot of value.

Don't forget the staff that's on duty during the times you're not there, particularly the night staff. Patients with Alzheimer's are often restless at night, so being on night duty is hardly a cushy job. Make sure that whatever gifts you provide are shared among all the shifts. If you bake cookies, make two batches, one to put out for those workers who are there when you visit and one for the next shift.

By the way, I'd also recommend making friends with the families of other residents in the facility. These people can act as your eyes and ears when you're not around, and you can do the same for them. This is particularly important if your loved one has a roommate, but even the families of other residents can be a good resource.

YOU AND YOUR CARE RECIPIENT'S DOCTOR

Because of the insurance situation in our country, whether yours is a private insurance fund, Medicare, or a combination of the two that pay for your care recipient's medical care, doctors today are forced to manage their time very carefully. Your job, therefore, is to get the most out of each doctor's visit, knowing that you usually cannot expect to get everything you want.

The first time your relationship with your care recipient's doctor will affect you is right at the beginning of the process of diagnosing Alzheimer's. It is vital that Alzheimer's be diagnosed as early as possible so that treatment can begin. However, figuring out what may be affecting an organ as complicated as the brain is time-consuming, and, if your doctor is a primary care physician, he or she is not a specialist in matters of brain functioning. So, no matter how much you and your care recipient love and trust this doctor, you have to consider from the very beginning that you might have to go elsewhere for medical attention, i.e. to a doctor who specializes in this area. (See Chapter 8 for a list of the type of specialists that treat Alzheimer's.) The truth is that more than 90 percent of Alzheimer's cases are not diagnosed as soon as they could be, so in the early stages, you are fighting an uphill battle to obtain the correct diagnosis, which, considering it is one you don't want to hear, will not seem like something you'll want to push for. And here's another factor: With more and more people reaching the ages when Alzheimer's is most prevalent, the medical world is going to have a hard time keeping up with the demand for diagnosis and treatment.

Even a specialist can allocate only so much time to you, so you must be fully prepared for each visit. You have to have as much down in writing as possible, including all the various changes in symptoms and behaviors that you've noticed since the last visit, a complete list of medications (as you might be seeing more than one doctor), and any reactions to those medications that have appeared. If you can send this list to the specialist ahead of time, great; if not, have it handy to give to the doctor. (Whether you send it ahead of time, or give it to the doctor, there's no insuring that the doctor will give it more than a cursory glance. That may be frustrating, but since the preparation of that list will help you ask the right questions, it's still worth doing.)

Making the most of the answers you do get is also going to present you with a hurdle. You might become upset at the doctor's first answer, which will keep you from paying attention to what else the doctor has to say. Or, the doctor's answer may prompt more questions, again distracting you. Thus, you have to have a way of recording the doctor's responses. It could be with pen and paper or on something more high-tech. It's good to have a way to retrieve this information later. (If you can bring a relative or friend along with you, that's all the better, as two sets of ears will make it more likely that you get everything down pat. You could even give this other person the main job of writing everything down, leaving you free to ask questions.)

On the one hand, you have to respect the doctor's time, but you have to balance that with the needs of your care recipient, so while you can't expect much chitchat, you do have to make sure that you have sufficient time to ask your most important questions. That's why your questions and concerns need to be written on a list and ranked according to importance. Also, keep in mind that you'll have to do this while trying to keep your care recipient as calm as possible in what may be a very upsetting situation for him or her. Let me repeat, if there is any way that you can bring along someone to help, do so. You may be able to handle most caregiving duties on your own, but this is one situation where the more attention you can give to communicating with the doctor, the better.

Just because doctors have time constraints doesn't mean they have an excuse not to give your care recipient the attention he or she deserves. So, don't be afraid of changing physicians if you think your loved one needs better treatment. However, this decision needs to be balanced by the level of expertise the doctor has. The better the doctor, the more patients he or she will have, and, thus, the more pressed for time he or she is likely to be. So if you've managed to get the best doctor for Alzheimer's treatment in your vicinity to take your care recipient on as a patient, you might end up having to give up more control than you would like. Of course, sometimes the very best physicians also have the best bedside manners, so don't assume that you'll be getting less than his or her full attention, because that might not be the case.

Also, don't ignore the rest of the doctor's staff. It could be that there are people on staff who have a lot to offer you, so talk to them and learn what you can. Having an ally in a doctor's office can pay off in the long run. Some nurses and other staff people may have more practical knowledge and be able to offer better advice than even the doctor.

What this chapter shows is that you face a dichotomy. On the one hand, you need help, but on the other, getting this help is going to cause you more work and require an additional skill set or two. What you need to be convinced of is that in the long run it's worth the effort. You're in this for the long haul, and so the preparations you make in the beginning to get the best help will definitely pay off in the end.

7

Helping Children and Grandchildren Cope

It's difficult enough for adults to grasp all the ramifications of Alzheimer's, so as you can imagine, it's quite a chasm for children to cross, young or teenaged. It's particularly hard if, in the case of early-onset Alzheimer's, it is a child's parent who is affected—but most of the time the child's close relative with Alzheimer's is a grandparent.

Because Alzheimer's progresses continually, it's important that you not hide from a child that this person he or she knows and loves is going to be going through dramatic changes. Younger children will often take a grandparent for granted, as someone who is there to love, without understanding that because of their age they won't be around forever. Therefore, it's vital that during the time when a grandparent can still interact with their grandchildren that they do so as much as possible. You want to make sure that the last image a child has of Grandma or Grandpa isn't just the one of them at their worst, but that instead those memories from the final days are well balanced against many other, more positive memories.

I know it's going to be tempting to keep the diagnosis of Alzheimer's secret from children, but since there is no cure and the child is going to see the changes taking place no matter what, it is better to be proactive than to try to cover up what is happening. Yes, long good-byes may be sadder, but rest assured that when these children become adults they will thank you for making them a full part of the transition time, before dementia sets in entirely.

Another reason to be open about what is happening is that there may be more than one grandchild involved in this process. You don't want an older child communicating the wrong message to a younger one. You want to control the family dynamics as best and as positively as you can, though it may not always be possible to have full control. If you are hiding what is going on, however, children will sense it anyway, and the outcome is then more likely to come out negatively, especially if it causes a child to be anxious or afraid.

By the way, this process is a two-way street. By making sure that children spend as much quality time with a grandparent as possible, this will also help to raise the grandparent's spirits in what are going to be very trying times. Whether it's a trip to Disneyland or a game of Go Fish, being with their grandchildren will help to take their minds off the fears surrounding their current situation. In fact, there is probably nothing that gives them more pleasure during this time period than being with children, so if this means missing school activities occasionally, or taking a season off from playing Little League, do all you can to keep this grand-parent together with his or her grandchildren as often as possible. Getting the child's cooperation is one reason why you have to explain to the child exactly what is transpiring. Let the child know that he or she is actually being a big help by spending time with Grandma or Grandpa and that helping to bolster their spirits is an important contribution.

There's something else you need to do when your children are with their grandparent: Document these moments. Take lots of pictures of Grandma reading a book to them, or shoot a ton of video of Grandpa taking them fishing. This way, they'll have mementos to support those wonderful memories. It is going to be difficult for a child to forget their grandparent's final days. But if later on you can put out a lot of pictures of them together in happier times, it will help reinforce the positive memories and downplay those that are better forgotten.

That's not to say that, once dementia advances, every second will be so bad that you won't want the children to have any memories of those times. Young children may be able to interact with their grandparent better than adults. If they can finger paint with Grandpa, this is an activity they'll both enjoy. Afterward, you can hang up their painting, so that the child has a visible reminder that Grandpa can be a lot of fun.

When an older person is a widow or widower, one thing they all miss is being touched, regardless of their mental state. We all need to be touched, but people who live alone usually miss this especially. Again, here young children can help to fill that void. Put on a video that the child enjoys and plop them in Grandma's lap so that they can watch together. Grandma may not care for what's being shown, but she'll treasure having a warm little body up against her.

Children who are slightly older may enjoy doing things for a grandparent that will help fill the time. You can have a fourth-grader read a simple book to their grandparent. This will serve many purposes. The child will feel good about being helpful, will be building up positive memories, and will be better able to keep the relationship going. If Grandma is always sitting in a corner by herself, she'll come to appear as a piece of furniture. By reading to Grandma, Grandma becomes more of a real, present person, even if she's not entirely sure who it is that is reading to her or what the story is about.

Children can help in other ways. If their grandparent needs help being fed, it's a chore they may be able to handle. A little girl might brush Grandma's hair, or put cream on her hands and arms. A little boy might be put in charge of reminding a grandparent to go to the toilet or change channels on the TV. If Grandpa is into sports, they could watch a game together.

The point is to be creative in finding ways of maintaining the connection so that both child and grandparent feel the benefits that can arise from such a relationship. The level of help a child can give will differ depending on age and personality, but regardless of age don't allow a child to lose all contact. Dealing with someone with dementia may not be the most pleasant of tasks, yet it's still a teachable moment for any child. It will help them to better understand that life isn't about only happy times. Having to deal with a grandparent with Alzheimer's will lead to personal growth and, overall, can be a positive experience if you help to pave the way for that outcome.

Of course, you'll have to address any fears that the child may have. For many children, this will be their first experience with either serious illness of disease. They'll need help in dealing with what is going on. There are plenty of children's books that deal with such topics, and I'd recommend looking through some and choosing the ones that you feel will help your child. Reading them together will allow you to address the topics raised in the book. If you are particularly under a lot of pressure due to the duties of raising a family, or perhaps working outside the home, as well as being a caregiver, perhaps you can assign someone else the role of helping children through this. It could be an older sibling, another grandparent, or an aunt or uncle.

The changes brought on by Alzheimer's won't happen overnight, but they can be significant over a relatively short period of time. If a child frequently spends time with their grandparent, they'll notice the changes, which will give them time to adapt. A grandchild who rarely sees a grandparent may have a bit more difficulty dealing with the severity of the change that has taken place, particularly if they haven't been together in a while. That's going to be especially true if their grandparent suddenly doesn't recognize them. For that reason, it's important to keep grandchildren in the loop as much as possible. Parents shouldn't hide news of the disease's progression. Yes, it would be better if they could be around their grandparent more often, but by keeping them fully informed, they'll be less shocked when they do see them.

Teens

I know a psychologist who did a study that showed that the whole idea of adolescence is a myth. In other societies, including in early American history, rebellion isn't part of a teen's life; instead, teens are often married and working at full-time jobs. It is mostly in modern Western societies where teens are required to remain in school, and thus not allowed to become full-fledged adults, where this rebellious attitude tends to develop. Nevertheless, teens in our society do have a unique status, and I can't wave a magic wand and make it go away. The fact that we encourage them to stay in school does artificially extend their childhood, but despite that, there are many teens who act as responsibly as adults, and in some cases more so.

My guess is that how you treat your teen on other life matters will carry over to how they react toward a grandparent with Alzheimer's. If your teen already helps out with chores and maybe even has a part-time job, he or she will more easily be integrated into the caregiving process. However, a teen who's never been given responsibilities beyond doing his or her homework is more likely to resent being asked to help out. Since I don't know your teens, I can't assume anything, so let me offer you some general suggestions on how your teen could be integrated into the care of their grandparent, especially if the teen and the grandparent are living under the same roof.

Because teens are capable of contributing a great deal toward caring for a grandparent, I would urge you to sit down with your teen and let him offer up a plan. Hopefully, he can come up with a schedule that will be helpful but not cramp his lifestyle too much. Of course, it's quite possible that the care of the grandparent places a very large burden on your family, especially financially, in which case teens in the family are going to have to kick in as much as possible, and the schedule is not going to be voluntary but rather practical. If that's the case, don't be afraid to use whatever tools are at your disposal, including a cautious degree of guilt, to get their full support.

The point is to treat your teen like an adult as much as possible, and in such a serious matter, I believe a teen will respond in an adult manner. But if you shoulder all the burden of what is happening and don't ask your teen to be a partner, there's every chance that a teen will shirk his or her responsibilities as a result of a combination of peer pressure (it's not cool to say you can't go out because you have to take care of a grandparent), the difficulties in taking care of someone with dementia, and the negative emotions the challenges inherent in the situation will cause your teen.

However, even a teen who volunteers to help can be prone to peer pressure. If all of his friends are going bowling, he's going to want to go too in order not to feel left out. So, a key word when it comes to getting teens to assist you is *consistency*. Many teens are very good at coming up with excuses. You must not give in, because once you start heading down that road, the excuses will come at a fast and furious pace. If a teen has promised to take care of Grandpa on Thursday afternoons after school, he must be held to that appointment, unless he knows in advance that he needs to alter the schedule, and then with proper notice changes can be made. But last-second excuses should not be acceptable.

It may be possible for a teen to pull a Tom Sawyer and get a friend to help. On the one hand, that may be okay, as having a peer to socialize with may make his or her assignment more palatable. But you have to be careful that this doesn't turn into a social visit, leaving the grandparent feeling abandoned. Since it's possible that this grandparent may not be able to report conduct that is inappropriate, you have to supervise to the best of your ability if a friend of your teen comes over, and I would limit it to only one. If the invited friend is one you don't particularly care for, then speak up. A bad influence in such a situation could spell real trouble.

On the one hand, I don't want to sound too negative when it comes to young people in this age group, while on the other, I know that peer pressure can propel them to act inappropriately. The bottom line is that helping to care for a grandparent with Alzheimer's can be what is called a "teachable moment." The teen can not only provide useful assistance, but can also learn some important life lessons. Learning to cope with adversity is a necessary skill. A teen who pitches in will come out stronger for the experience. So, whether you feel your teen is mostly responsible or mostly irresponsible, I would encourage you to make him or her part of the caregiving team. They have a lot to provide in terms of manpower and love and can learn a lot from the experience, so you should do all you can to make them an active participant.

There is also the question of the teen's feelings about the changes he or she witnesses in their grandparent. Many teens have been around their grandparents all their life, so this is someone they know well. While adults can't be fully prepared to deal with someone with Alzheimer's, teens will be even less so. Some may be afraid to show their real emotions, while others may actually become hysterical. Since a teen's emotions may be on a bit of a roller coaster ride as their own hormones go up and down, exactly how they'll react on a day-to-day basis may be unpredictable. However, that shouldn't change their overall duty to help out. If a teen says, "It freaks me out to see Grandma like this," the teen has to be made to understand that it freaks everyone out. Let your teen know that this is an experience that you'd prefer not to have as well, but explain to them the importance of family cooperation and instill in them a sense of duty, both of which will stand them in good stead for the rest of their life. Doing chores that you'd rather not do is part of growing up, and the more a teen wants to be treated as an adult, the more he or she is going to have to adapt to this situation.

To encourage a teen to act more like an adult by playing an important role in the care of his or her grandparent, you should allow your teen a little more freedom at other times. If a teen is showing that he or she is very responsible when it comes to taking care of a grandparent, especially one with Alzheimer's, which is not an easy task, you might consider giving your son or daughter more freedom in other matters as an acknowledgment that they are showing the maturity that warrants more privileges.

Remind your son or daughter of any age that he or she is also helping you. Don't try to hide how hard this situation is on you and your spouse. When parents have difficulties, whether financial or health or relationship-wise, the tendency is often to "protect" the child. However, children often sense something is wrong and may think that they are at fault, so at least a certain amount of honesty is the better approach. And, when it comes to a close relative with Alzheimer's, well, that isn't something that's easily swept under the rug. It's better to be honest with your child and work to allay their fears than to cover up a situation that in the near future is going to make itself known, no matter what.

Danger Signs

Having a significant other who's afflicted with a disease like Alzheimer's is definitely going to be upsetting to your children, whatever their age. That they become sad or upset is understandable. But there are sometimes indications that they may be more impacted by the situation emotionally than may be healthy. If their behavior changes in any significant ways, speak to them about it. Be alert for major difference in sleep habits, a decrease in grades, a change in their social life, desiring to spend more or less time with friends, or wanting to be alone. I've been saying here that children need to be part of the process, but that doesn't mean that every child is capable of handling Alzheimer's at such close range. You might even note a difference is how siblings react. If one child is showing signs of having a serious problem dealing with a grandparent with Alzheimer's—let's say his or her grades suddenly nosedive—you may have to take steps to protect this child. Maybe some counseling will work. Or, maybe this child would benefit from a break by going on sleepovers or spending more time with friends.

If a child who seems to be having a difficult time with this situation won't talk to you about it, seek help. Help could come from another family member, like a trusted aunt or uncle. Your child may feel that he or she can't tell you their real feelings because they know how badly you feel, but they may have a strong need to communicate. And, if this behavior continues, don't hesitate to seek professional help.

Having a grandparent change to such an extent that they no longer recognize family members is going to have a negative effect on every one of you. How could it not? How your children react is not insignificant, so be sensitive to how they're acting. If the patient is really out of it and having him or her in the home is having quite a negative impact, that might push you toward sending the care recipient to a facility earlier than you had planned—and this in turn might offer a positive change that would be good for your entire family, as well as for you.

I mentioned earlier that a child might benefit from speaking to another, older relative. The same could be true for you, though the relative wouldn't need to be older, just an adult. Sometimes, you really can't see the forest for the trees. You may really be too close to your children, especially if you're under stress, to clearly assess how they're acting. So, if you have any doubts, or even if you don't, speak to someone who is not so closely involved with the situation and see what they think. Your elderly parent is obviously very important to you, but at this stage in their lives, your children come first. You don't want to coddle them, but you also don't want to push them so hard that they break under the strain.

PART TWO:

STANDING ON THE SHOULDERS OF GIANTS

8

Treating Alzheimer's

At the beginning of this book, I told you that I am neither a medical doctor nor an Alzheimer's specialist. But one cannot write a book about caring for those who have Alzheimer's without also offering up at least some information about the disease itself, as well as offering advice from others who are involved in the medical care of this disease. So, in this second part of the book, I'm going to pass on to you the information I think is important for you to have.

As we age, our mental function diminishes. That shouldn't surprise anyone, as the rest of our body starts to slowly decline from its peak performance once we get past our twenties. Once we hit our fifties, the changes become more and more noticeable. But most of these changes don't prevent us from going forward with our lives, even if we must do so a bit more cautiously. (That I had to give up skiing a few years ago still bothers me!) As to our brain functioning, almost everyone notices at a certain stage in life that trying to recall certain pieces of information, like the name of that person walking up to you at a cocktail party, can be difficult. The cutesy term for this is "having a senior moment." We all have them. I certainly do at age eighty-four, but in my case, and in the case of most people, it's not a very dramatic shift and doesn't really interfere with my day-to-day activities. However, that's not true for the millions of people who suffer from dementia.

Dementia is defined as a loss of brain function that causes problems with our memory, thinking, and behavior. In the days when medicine was less informed about dementia, it was usually labeled as senility. Today, we know there are many causes of dementia, one of which is a disease called

Alzheimer's. The disease is named after Dr. Alois Alzheimer, the doctor who discovered certain changes in the brain of a patient he autopsied, way back in 1906.

It is impossible to say for certain whether someone has Alzheimer's without doing an autopsy of the brain after the person has died, though nowadays an MRI might detect signs of possible Alzheimer's, and, in the near future, brain scans will be able to detect damage occurring within the brain long before any symptoms materialize. When scientists look at the brain tissue of people who have had Alzheimer's, they find a variety of evidence, including "neurofibrillary tangles" (twisted fragments of protein within nerve cells that clog up the cell), "neuritic plaques" (abnormal clusters of dead and dying nerve cells, other brain cells, and protein) and "senile plaques" (areas where products of dying nerve cells have accumulated around protein). It seems that in people susceptible to Alzheimer's, a genetic trait doesn't allow them to put the brakes on the process of plaque buildup. But while the patient is still living, a specialist in dementia can usually make the diagnosis based on behavioral evidence.

There are two basic types of Alzheimer's, early-onset, which means the person begins showing symptoms before the age of sixty, and late-onset, which is much more common and which begins after the age of sixty. The older you are, the more likely it is that you will get Alzheimer's. In fact, the instance of Alzheimer's doubles every five years beyond age sixty-five. There are an estimated 5.4 million people living with Alzheimer's in the United States, and Alzheimer's is the sixth-leading cause of death in this country, and, of the top ten causes, it is the only disease that currently cannot be prevented, slowed, or cured. Of those with dementia, the cause in 60 to 80 percent of these cases is considered to be Alzheimer's. (Remember, there is no way to know for sure whether Alzheimer's is the cause until after the person has died, and then only if an autopsy is done.) Some of the other causes include vascular dementia, Parkinson's disease, Creutzfeldt-Jakob disease, and Huntington's disease, as well as a whole laundry list of diseases with various acronyms that I won't bore you with. However, interestingly enough, it's also possible that what may appear to be dementia is not dementia at all.

IT MIGHT NOT BE DEMENTIA

Some of the symptoms of dementia, like memory loss, can be triggered by other conditions that are treatable and reversible. Some medications to treat conditions such as high blood pressure can cause memory loss or other signs of what appears to be some malfunction of the brain. The same is true of kidney failure, depression, and anemia. (The latter causes the brain to get less oxygen and so perform more poorly.) A lack of sleep can cause symptoms and so can the medications to help one fall asleep. A small stroke, often caused by diabetes, which is very common among older people, can be behind the symptoms. Surgery can sometimes cause memory loss. Approximately 30 percent of those who have open-heart surgery suffer from some memory loss (and for many of these, it is not reversible, though it also doesn't continue to worsen). Chemotherapy can also affect the brain. And, if someone is suffering from hearing loss or has vision problems that haven't been addressed, what may appear to be memory loss might be nothing more than an inability to process certain information in the first place. For example, if an older person can't hear someone's name, naturally she won't remember it later. Another very common occurrence is that a person may be affected by several of these factors at the same time, multiplying the effect.

So as you can see, deciding for yourself (like self-diagnosis) that certain symptoms are Alzheimer's can be a big mistake, particularly if information about these symptoms is withheld from a doctor who is treating the patient for some other ailment. If you notice any symptoms of what may be dementia in someone else or in yourself, don't delay in seeing a doctor. (See the Eleven Warning Signs later in this chapter.) This is especially important if the cause is something other than Alzheimer's, because the underlying problem may not only be treatable, but may cause other damage if it is not treated.

If Alzheimer's is the cause of someone's symptoms, it's also important to see a doctor, as the medications that can be prescribed to slow the disease might give the patient added time to live an almost normal life. So, whatever you do, don't make the mistake of diagnosing what's happening as Alzheimer's and just giving up. (By the way, if you have a strong genetic disposition towards Alzheimer's, you may want to begin taking medications against the disease long before you show any signs of it. This idea is only now being given serious consideration in the medical field, but if you think you might be a candidate for such early preventive treatment, ask your doctor any time after your fortieth birthday.)

At this point I'd like to quote further from the article written by Robin Leckie (mentioned earlier in the book), as I think it's quite appropriate:

It seems like just a few days, not three years, since I called to my wife, asking her to sit beside me while I shared some news. The winter sun was filling the room with warmth, and rainbow colors streamed through the stained-glass window. I had just returned from a doctor's appointment and now what I had expected for some time had been confirmed—I had Alzheimer's.

Earlier, as I returned home that morning, I remember feeling somehow relieved, even though this was what I had anticipated. All those isolated moments of memory loss, confusion, and indecision now had a reason—in the same way as when we have a complaint and make a doctor's appointment and part of us hopes the complaint will still be there when we arrive. I was the same person before the appointment as after; I still looked the same. But now I knew I was faced with an uncertain future.

No one wants to have Alzheimer's, but as Robin so admirably demonstrates, if you've been struggling with what you're worried might be dementia, you'll be better off with a diagnosis than remaining in the dark.

Playing Doctor

Sometimes it may be obvious to a medical professional what is going on with a patient, and sometimes it won't be. So if someone you know is given a diagnosis of, say, depression, and this doesn't make sense to you, don't be afraid to question such a diagnosis. Seek out a second, third, or fourth opinion, if necessary. Understandably, no one wants to hear a diagnosis of Alzheimer's, but as I've said, since the correct medication may slow down the progress of the disease, the sooner you discover the truth, the better.

The difficulty for you is how to navigate these waters, given your lack of real medical knowledge. You are certainly not capable of telling the difference between depression in a loved one (or in yourself for that matter) and the early signs of dementia. And, given how scary a diagnosis of dementia is, are you really going to be motivated to find the truth? Pursuing a second opinion can involve a number of costs, in terms of time, money, and energy, which make going on a wild goose chase problematic. I would suggest asking close relatives for their advice. Whether or not they can actually help you, I don't know, but by asking the opinions of people who know the person in question, you may reach a consensus.

At the very least, if you've involved other people in the decision-making process, you'll feel less guilty if your intuition is incorrect.

There's another reason to ask others who know your loved one what they think. Sometimes, the signs of Alzheimer's are more pronounced in certain circumstances. Let's say your husband loves to play cards, but you don't, so you never play with him. His friends may have begun to notice some definite changes in his playing abilities that you would never know about. They might not come to you with this information on their own, but if you ask them, they probably will tell you the truth. So, rather than hide your suspicions, if your loved one is at the stage where he or she hasn't yet been diagnosed, start asking questions.

While the detectable symptoms of Alzheimer's generally don't appear until after age sixty, the disease actually takes a long time to develop. Damage to the brain can begin ten to twenty years before any symptoms make themselves known. At the moment, that window of opportunity doesn't offer any ways to stop the disease's progress, but hopefully one day, early detection might allow doctors to medically intervene before too much damage is done. There are drugs available today that have a limited ability to do that. (More on these drugs later.) Thus, if you suspect that someone you know has the very beginnings of dementia, don't put off seeing a doctor. Obviously, it's not a diagnosis anyone wants to hear, but if hearing it sooner allows you to slow down its progress, why would you ever wait to get an evaluation?

ELEVEN WARNING SIGNS

Most of you reading this book are dealing with someone who has already received a diagnosis of Alzheimer's, so I'm not going to go into the eleven warning signs too deeply, but I also don't want to leave this information out of the book, so here they are in brief:

1. Memory loss that disrupts daily life, especially asking the same question over and over.

2. Challenges in planning or problem solving, such as no longer being able to follow a recipe or taking much longer than usual to do routine tasks.

3. Difficulty completing familiar tasks, like driving to a destination the person knows well or forgetting how to play a simple game.

4. Confusion with time or place, so that they may not be able to keep track of what day it is or where they are.

5. Trouble understanding visual images or spatial relationships, so that activities like driving or reading may become difficult.

6. New problems with speaking and writing that go beyond just forgetting the occasional word. Some may be unable to continue a conversation.

7. Losing things and not being able to find them because they can't remember enough to retrace their steps.

8. Decreased or poor judgment, particularly over money matters, but this may also be visible via changes in grooming habits.

9. Withdrawal from work or social activities, often because of embarrassment.

10. Changes in mood and personality. They may be moody, become suspicious even of people they know, and become easily upset.

11. Finally, here's a new symptom that has recently been discovered: an inability to tell truth from untruth, including everything from outright lies to mere sarcasm.

One reason to become familiar with these signs, even if the person in your care has already been diagnosed, is that, as a caregiver, you're a source of knowledge for friends, relatives, and neighbors on the subject of Alzheimer's. You're likely to be asked questions, so knowing these eleven signs will probably come in handy.

The Stages

When I began writing this book, there were said to be seven stages to Alzheimer's. But in the middle of the writing process, an announcement was made by the National Institute on Aging and the Alzheimer's Association that redefined the stages. The reason behind this was to reflect the fact that Alzheimer's begins to develop much earlier than was previously thought, and there are important reasons to recognize this. The newly reported first stage is one where changes are occurring in the brain but there are no apparent symptoms. At this stage, the person has no idea that Alzheimer's is developing within the brain and the disease is beginning to go on the offensive. The second stage can be described as early Alzheimer's, when there are some symptoms but the victim can still function on his or her own to a great extent. The third stage is when dementia has set in, and the person is no longer fully functional.

Why is it important to give greater recognition to the first stage when there are no symptoms? (I know I'm repeating this message, but since there's no cure, this aspect of Alzheimer's bears repeating several times.) It is important because if Alzheimer's can be detected early enough, either existing drugs or new drugs yet to be developed may be able to thwart the disease from doing major damage. Often, by the time either the person with Alzheimer's or his or her relatives or friends notice changes significant enough to warrant sending this person for a medical diagnosis, it is too late to do much about arresting the course of the disease. Thus, early testing will become more and more important, and therefore it is vital that the public be made aware of the importance of early detection.

BASIC TESTS

The American Academy of Neurology recommends two basic tests for early signs of Alzheimer's:

Mini Mental Status Exam: A short, untimed test that quantifies cognitive function and screens for cognitive loss by testing a person's orientation, attention, calculation, recall, and language and motor skills. There are eleven sections in the test, including naming common objects, writing a sentence, and copying a design of two intersecting shapes. Patients receive one point for each correct answer.

Memory Impairment Screen: A four-item recall test that assesses memory impairment. Patients are given the names of one item in each of the following categories: animal, city, vegetable, and musical instrument. After a short delay, the individuals are asked to recite the four items in any order. If the patient misses an item, the physician cues the individual by telling him or her the category.

The other key message that these scientists want to convey is that memory loss is not necessarily the first indication of Alzheimer's. Mood changes or problems with language, spatial perception, or reasoning might also be indications of the onset of Alzheimer's, and the more people are aware of these signs, the more likely it is that early detection will occur.

113

There are physical markers that the medical world is just now learning how to detect. As this aspect of Alzheimer's treatment is developed, it will be possible to screen more people at an earlier age with good results. Those with a family history of Alzheimer's, for example, would need to be screened early, similar to how patients with a family history of breast cancer are screened early.

There remains a lot of work to be done. One third of those who develop some of the physical markers of Alzheimer's, such as amyloid plaques, never develop the disease. However, diagnostic testing, such as X-rays, is important to employ in early detection efforts, as two thirds of those with these markers do develop Alzheimer's.

While I certainly agree with how important it is to publicize the message that early diagnosis is key, I also think that the old seven stages serve a purpose to those who know that they or a loved one has Alzheimer's. When communicating with the physician taking care of the patient, for example, it can be useful to use these stages as a way of indicating where on the Alzheimer's scale a person currently falls. So, while these seven stages may soon fall out of favor, at this time they should be used to whatever degree seems valuable.

The Stages of Alzheimer's

The old Stage One is the same as the new Stage One, as there are no visible signs of impairment or obvious symptoms, but damage is taking place inside the brain. Since there are no signs of this damage, the ordinary tests that a doctor might use, such as the most common battery of memory tests, won't reveal anything. However, X-rays or brain scans might reveal physical damage occurring within the brain. As already noted, such damage may not end up leading to Alzheimer's, but perhaps, combined with other factors, like the carrying of certain genes, treatment with drugs might be initiated as a precautionary measure. So, if you notice changes in yourself or a loved one that seem minor, don't ignore them. It's better to be tested and find nothing than not be tested and risk further damage if the disease goes unchecked.

In Stage Two, there is very mild cognitive decline. The person may say to himself or herself that it's becoming harder and harder to remember certain things, but no one else around the person would be able to detect any differences. What you might notice is a change in personality or behavior as this person reacts to the changes he or she is feeling. Again, rather than ignore them, or allow this person to shrug them off, try to explore what is occurring.

Let me repeat here that some of these changes may be the result of another medical problem, one that is treatable, so this is another reason to see a doctor, even if you are afraid the diagnosis might be Alzheimer's.

In Stage Three, those around the person will begin to notice changes. The person will have noticeable difficulty coming up with a word or someone's name, even if they've just been introduced. If the person is still employed, he or she may have difficulties with tasks that were once easy to perform. Planning and organizing skills weaken or disappear. The person will lose track of objects, even those that are valuable.

MILD COGNITIVE IMPAIRMENT (MCI)

Stage Four has been labeled Mild Cognitive Impairment, and the symptoms at this point will allow for a diagnosis of Alzheimer's. This stage would now be called Stage Two. In this stage, forgetfulness becomes more apparent. Tasks that require mathematical skills, like paying bills, may become difficult or impossible to perform. Medical tests will include using those skills, such as asking the person to count backwards from one hundred by increments of seven. Accompanying these changes in memory skills will be changes in the person's emotional behavior. He or she is likely to become moody or withdrawn, especially in social settings.

MODERATELY SEVERE COGNITIVE DECLINE

Moderately Severe Cognitive Decline is the label for Stage Five. While someone at this stage can still feed himself or herself and go to the toilet on their own, they are going to need help in many other ways. They won't remember what day it is, or what month it is, and they will need help dressing in clothing that is appropriate for the season. They'll become confused about where they are. They won't remember important information about themselves such as their address, phone number, or what high school they attended.

SEVERE COGNITIVE DECLINE

Stage Six is considered to be Severe Cognitive Decline, though this is actually mid-stage Alzheimer's disease, as the patient may continue to decline for some time. As the patient's memory continues to worsen, they will need more and more help in performing everyday activities. They'll remember their own name but may have difficulty remembering that of their spouse or daily caregiver. They can distinguish between people they know and don't know but may not know who each individual is. They will lose the ability to dress themselves, forgetting to take their clothes off and putting on their pajamas over their clothes, for example. They will require help using the toilet, as they're likely to forget to wipe themselves or flush. Or, they may forget to go to the toilet altogether and lose control of their bowel or bladder.

Their sleep pattern may change so that they'll be too restless at night to sleep and then sleep during the day. Their personalities may also change so that they may become suspicious, thinking that their caregiver is an imposter, or they may experience delusions. They may also exhibit compulsive repetitive behavior, like handwringing or rubbing certain articles over and over. There is also a tendency to wander off, which is why constant supervision at this stage becomes necessary. (I'll include tips on how to handle some of these behaviors in the next chapter.)

THE FINAL STAGE

Stage Seven is called Late-stage Alzheimer's or Very Severe Cognitive Decline. In this stage, the patient is going to need help with everything, including eating and going to the toilet. They won't say very much, maybe a word or two if you try to initiate conversation. They may also lose the ability to smile, to sit without support, and to hold their heads up. Reflexes become abnormal. Muscles grow rigid, and swallowing is impaired.

Of course, there are no clear lines of demarcation between these stages. Some people with dementia exhibit all of the symptoms of a certain stage, while others may not. Is it important for you to know the stages? The first and last stages are particularly important. As I've been saying, the earlier you spot Alzheimer's, the more helpful the current drug therapy may be. Also, you won't want to waste a second making the proper legal and financial plans if your loved one appears to be developing Alzheimer's. (See Chapter 12 for more information.) As your loved one moves into the last stages, you are probably approaching the time when you are going to have to send your loved one to a facility. Some of the factors in that decision will be entirely personal, but recognizing that he or she is in the latter stages will be a consideration.

PERSONAL STAGES

Apart from the official stages, you are going to find that your care recipient will go through some personal stages. In other words, there are stages that some Alzheimer's patients undergo, but not all patients progress in the same way. For example, your mother may become very argumentative. Or your father may become paranoid and accuse you of stealing his belongings. Not every patient with Alzheimer's exhibits such behavior, but for those who do, whether this development happens during Stage Three, Four, or Five is irrelevant to you. All that matters is that for a time you're going to have to find a way to deal with this "stage," and the key phrase here is "for a time."

Some of these personal stages can be quite difficult for you to handle. If your mother is constantly blaming you for things that you've done or not done and there's no truth to these accusations, you are going to want to argue with her, yet that is useless, as she is suffering from a delusion. Instead, you have to not take her accusations to heart and try to divert her attention to something else. Now, if this behavior were to become permanent and go on for years, this would be hard to take. But in most cases, it's just a stage your care recipient is going through, much the way toddlers go through stages. At some point, this behavior will change. I can't promise you that it will be a change for the better, but just knowing that a change is coming and you'll no longer be accused of stealing, for example, will make hearing these charges again and again more bearable.

WHAT CAN BE DONE

As I've said repeatedly, there is no cure for Alzheimer's, but if it's caught early enough, there are drugs that can slow the process down. In fact, in talking to people about this subject, someone reported having an uncle who was diagnosed with early-onset Alzheimer's, and after being put on these medications the uncle reported that he felt more mental clarity than he had in years. I hope for his sake the effects of these drugs last for him, but as I said, in general, all that can be hoped for is a slowdown in the progression of the disease, and the difference between being on such medication or not will usually not seem to make much of a difference in the symptoms of your loved one. (Again, if you believe you are geneti-cally inclined to get Alzheimer's, being put on medication long before you show any signs of the disease may delay the onset.)

To date, the drugs that are being used are prescribed in what is called off-label use, meaning the drugs were developed for some other medical reason, but have been found to help with Alzheimer's. With an ever-growing need, and thus market, the pharmaceutical industry is busy trying to come up with drugs that will specifically target the symptoms of Alzheimer's. Hopefully, positive developments will happen sooner rather than later.

Since there are different symptoms that come with Alzheimer's, there are different drugs available that may be effective in treating some or all of them. The main symptom is, of course, memory loss, and right now there are two types of drugs that have been approved by the Food and Drug Administration with regards to memory loss: cholinesterase inhibitors (Aricept, Exelon, Razadyne, Cognex) and memantine (Namenda), which treat the cognitive symptoms (memory loss, confusion, and problems with thinking and reasoning) of Alzheimer's disease. These drugs may help the brain to continue to communicate within its cells, thus stem-ming the damage caused by Alzheimer's. Some doctors prescribe only one or both together. Some doctors may also add high dosages of Vitamin E. (While writing this book, I found an article in a medical publication that said that memantine was no more effective than a placebo. As we all know, the science of medicine seems to change all the time and it is very difficult for a lay person to comprehend exactly what is going on, yet we all have a responsibility to try to understand because there doesn't seem to be one path to follow. So, you can either trust your doctor and hope for the best, or you can do your own research and ask a lot of questions. See the Appendix for websites that will help you out if you follow the latter approach.)

You need to understand how these drugs work to be able to have a good picture of your care recipient's overall level of treatment. Since you're ultimately in charge, it's up to you to make sure that the person in your care is getting the best that modern medicine has to offer. But there are also aspects of drug therapy that you need to keep at the back of your mind. First of all, understand that drug therapy does not work for every Alzheimer's patient. In fact, these drugs have been found to work in less than half of those to whom they are administered. And the effects may be so limited that you won't even notice a difference, or the effects may be short-lived, so that a drug slows down the progress of the disease, but only for a limited period of time.

The point I want to make is that drugs are not a panacea. They can be useful, but in the end, your loved one is not going to escape the full ravages of the disease. I don't want you to place your hopes in the idea that the currently available drugs are going to rescue you, because that will only lead to disappointment. You don't want to get too excited by any progress you see, you don't want to become complacent about the preparations you need to make, and you don't want to live in a fantasy world that is one day going to come crashing down. Why not? Picture yourself in a hot air balloon sailing over some beautiful countryside. You're enjoying the view, but you know that you only have so much gas in your tank. If you fly too high up, so that when you run out of gas you're thousands of feet in the air, you're going to come crashing down. But if you're only a few hundred feet up, you can make a gentle, controlled descent when the time comes.

If you take a realistic view of what drugs can do for you and your loved one, you can enjoy the extra time you'll have at a lower stage of Alzheimer's, but your world won't come to an end if or when the drugs prove ineffective. If you can keep your care recipient under your roof for an extra six months, that's a wonderful plus, and just accept it as that, rather than getting angry at the drug for failing to completely halt the progress of the disease. Hopefully, the day will come when drugs prove more effective, but in the meantime try to recognize their limitations.

DRUG THERAPY

As mentioned, there are two types of drugs. The cholinesterase inhibitors are used in the early stages of the disease. Your brain naturally produces a chemical messenger, acetylcholine, and in patients with Alzheimer's, the production of this chemical decreases, which leads to memory loss. The cholinesterase inhibitors both increase the production of this chemical and increase its effectiveness. However, as the brain produces less and less acetycholine, the effect of the drug is reduced and eventually stops altogether, which is why these drugs work only in the early to mid-stages. Which type of cholinesterase is going to be right for your care recipient depends. Some may work better or have fewer side effects on a particular individual than others. So, if you're caring for someone who is using this drug, you'll have to monitor them as best as you can and make a detailed report to the prescribing physician so that a decision can be made whether or not to stay with a particular inhibitor or make a switch. Since the person in your care cannot communicate adequately, it is going to be up to you to maintain a steady flow of information between yourself and the doctor. Feel free to ask questions, and, if necessary, obtain a second opinion.

Memantine is a drug prescribed to patients with later stages of Alzheimer's, though often it is not substituted for a cholinesterase inhibitor but rather given as an additional drug. Again, you're going to be the one most likely to notice whether this drug is having a beneficial effect, especially in light of any ill effects it might have. Somebody is going to have to weigh the pros and cons, and if you spend the most time with the patient, then your opinion will count the most.

Bear in mind that since the most these drugs can do is slow down the rate of the brain's deterioration, it can be difficult to say for certain whether or not they are helping. If the side effects seem to outweigh the benefits and you and the doctor decide to stop giving the patient medication, but then you notice that the patient is starting to deteriorate rapidly in terms of memory loss after the drug has been stopped, don't hesitate to call the doctor and ask to resume the medication. It's understandable that since you don't have any medical training, you may hesitate to make such decisions, but the fact is that no doctor or scientist can predict exactly how these medications may act upon a specific patient. Since in this case you know the patient best, your input carries considerable weight, and don't hesitate to throw your weight around if it means that the person under your care will be getting the best possible treatment.

LATEST EFFORTS

Scientists are working on an assortment of other medications and treatments that will either prevent Alzheimer's or slow down its progress significantly once it is diagnosed, but these are still on the horizon. One that seemed promising had some serious side effects that made it impractical. On the other hand, I read about the concept of using electronic brain stimulation, which has worked to some extent with Parkinson's disease, on people with Alzheimer's, though this is still being tested.

One change that is on the horizon is that soon doctors will be able to perform a brain scan that will be able to distinguish the type of damage associated with Alzheimer's. Since there is no cure, there are some people who are not going to want to know. But as I've been saying, finding out sooner gives you more time to prepare. It's going to be a tough decision whether or not to go forward with this test, but I think the best choice, especially if a doctor recommends it, is to go forward.

DRUG ALTERNATIVES

I'm going to present more about what you can do to help your care recipient in the next chapter, but let me at least mention here that someone with Alzheimer's can often be helped with alternative treatments such as aromatherapy, yoga, pet therapy, massage therapy, etc. You may be skeptical about this, but such therapies have been tested in clinical settings and have been found to be helpful. So, don't skip reading about this in the next chapter.

DOCTOR'S VISITS

I've explained that because you spend so much time with your care recipient, and because he or she won't be able to communicate adequately, you're going to be the point person at each doctor's visit. (If you need to use someone else to perform this task, you're going to have to write down a very complete report on the state of your charge, both physically and mentally, as well as a list of questions to ask.) In order to make these doctor's visits as fruitful as possible, the following are some tips that I've gathered from various sources. (And polls show that most caregivers follow such suggestions, though there are still far too many who do not, which I think is a mistake.)

1. If the person in your care doesn't have a lot of patience, try to schedule appointments when there is less of a chance of having to endure a long wait. Don't hesitate to ask the receptionist when that might be.

2. In case there is a wait, be prepared. Many Alzheimer's patients can be distracted with food or drink, so bring some cookies and juice (or whatever they like best and is on their diet). Also, bring any activities that might entertain them. A portable DVD player with headphones might work for some.

3. If your care recipient is very difficult when taken out of the house for a doctor's visit, see if you can find a doctor who will come to your house. They do exist, and there are even dentists who make house calls.

4. Bring a detailed list of everything your loved one takes in terms of drugs and supplements. Medications are certainly the most important (and you can bring the actual pill containers so that you can be absolutely certain of the names and dosages), but vitamins and other supplements need to be on that list, and in what amounts. If your loved one has any health problems, it wouldn't be a bad idea to describe to their doctor their basic diet, because an allergy might be the cause of a problem.

    Tip: If you keep a daily log of all the medications and supplements you give your loved one, not only will that serve as a list to bring to your doctor, but it will also help you to be certain that all medications have been given every day. You can download from alz.org sample forms of the various logs that you might keep, such as a medication log and appointment log.

5. You also should make a list of any health issues, so that you don't forget to ask the right questions. Your list should be in the order of most important first, just in case your doctor has to cut the visit short, or your loved one is acting in a manner that means you can't stay. That way, you'll at least get your most important questions answered. If you want to type them up and give them to the doctor, that's OK too. (Many doctors will accept such lists via fax ahead of time, though rarely via e-mail because of malpractice issues.)

6. If this is an early visit, where a diagnosis is still being made, you definitely should bring a family history of the various conditions that your loved one may have inherited, and not just dementia, but all diseases, as this will help the doctor in making his or her diagnosis. If you don't know the family medical history all that well, ask any siblings or your aunts and uncles to fill in any gaps in your knowledge. A good medical history is an important tool to a doctor, and it's something only you can provide.

7. The main way that the doctor is going to be able to measure the progress of the disease is by getting as clear a picture as possible of

what's happening on a day-to-day basis. So, you should keep track of any changes in behavior or eating habits or anything else that seems to change. You should make note both of day-to-day changes and any particular incidents that might have taken place; for example, if your loved one had been able to go to the toilet by him or herself and no longer can, or if he or she became lost while taking his or her daily walk in the neighborhood.

8. If your loved one is taking medication, make note of any side effects that you suspect are being caused by the medication, like an upset stomach. Your doctor may prescribe a different medication that will be just as effective but won't cause this side effect.

9. Many people have a hard time remembering exactly what the doctor said after they leave the office. It's not your brain that's going, it's just that you are a bit nervous. It happens to lots of people, so bring a pad and pen, or even use your phone to record what the doctor says. Later on, you'll be glad you did.

10. If your loved one can answer questions, make sure that you sit in a place so that when the doctor is speaking to your loved one, you're in the doctor's line of sight. This will enable you to communicate silently with the doctor, with a nod or shake of your hand, as that will help the doctor to better understand what is going on at home.

11. Your doctor might not be able to help you solve every problem that you might run into while taking care of someone with dementia, but he or she might be a good source of referrals to other people or organizations that can offer help in these other areas, especially if he or she is a specialist and treats many people with dementia. So, don't be afraid to ask about non-medical issues.

12. Remember that your doctor is your main ally in this role you've taken on as caregiver. As your loved one hits various stages of the disease, your doctor should be able to provide valuable support. For example, if your loved one is in the early stages and is still driving, but you strongly believe he or she shouldn't be on the road, ask your doctor to back you up. Having the doctor say that driving is forbidden will make it easier on you when you need to take away the keys. (In six states, doctors are mandated by law to tell the Department of Motor Vehicles if they believe a patient is no longer

fit to drive, and the American Medical Association recommends to all of its members that they do so; therefore, you should have a ready ally in this respect.) In the latter stages, your doctor can help you make the decision of when it's time to send your loved one to a facility, so that the decision doesn't fall solely on your shoulders.

Tip: If your next doctor's visit is weeks away and you notice a sudden change in your loved one's health, don't wait for your scheduled appointment—call your doctor and make a new one.

Where Else to Go for Help

You probably went to your family doctor, or primary care physician as they're now called, when you first noticed that something was wrong. At some point, however, you may need a specialist in order to make sure that you're getting the best possible care for your loved one. The following are some specialists that you might want to consider:

- A **Geriatric Nurse Practitioner**, or GNP, is a nurse who has been certified by the American Nurses Credentialing Center, a certification that requires the nurse to receive a master's degree. Such nurses have a thorough knowledge of all the medical and behavioral issues your loved one might encounter and can make an excellent substitute when you cannot see your doctor.

- A **Geriatrician** is a medical doctor who has taken additional training in treating older adults. If you have one available to you, your loved one's geriatrician will probably be the main doctor he or she will be seeing for treatment.

- A **Geriatric Psychiatrist** has taken special courses in geriatrics and can both evaluate your loved one and prescribe medication. Having such a doctor as part of the team taking care of your loved one may prove essential, as behavioral issues are bound to crop up, and having the right person to help you will be crucial.

- A **Gerontologist** is not a medical doctor but has had special training so that he or she can lead support groups and help in the care of those with early-stage Alzheimer's.

- A **Geropsychologist** is a psychologist with the training and experience to deal with the mental health challenges of older people.

- A **Neurologist** is a medical doctor who specializes in certain diseases, including Alzheimer's and Parkinson's, as well as the aftermath of strokes. Because these diseases tend to hit the elderly, many have special training for this population, though not all do.

- A **Neuropsychologist** has had special training in the way the brain affects behavior and so is able to run tests to diagnose Alzheimer's and to judge the stage of the disease.

Alternative Medicine

Alzheimer's must be treated by a doctor of medicine, but that doesn't mean that others in the healthcare profession can't also be of service. Nutritionists can assist with ailments, such as constipation and digestive issues, and may offer guidance on the course and dosage of a vitamin regimen. There are those that believe vitamins, particularly B12, can help with Alzheimer's (for more on this subject, read the book *Could It Be B12?*). There have also been some studies that show Vitamin D may be helpful. If your loved one is suffering from backaches or other pains, a chiropractor may be of assistance. And, of course, massage therapy can help your loved one to feel more relaxed. (I love massages and have at least one a week.)

Acupuncture is known to have positive effects on the nervous system, and since agitation, anxiety, and depression are major problems among those with Alzheimer's, you may choose to reach out to an acupuncturist. I am far from an expert in this area, but if it's possible that your loved one might find some relief, and not become too agitated by the treatment, why not consider it?

As I mentioned earlier, if your alternative therapy route involves taking some sort of supplement, you must inform your doctor. You don't have to say why you are giving your loved one some specific vitamin or herb, but since such products could interfere with the way any pharmaceutical medication works, your doctor needs to be informed. For a treatment where nothing is ingested, like chiropractic manipulation or acupuncture, you need not tell your doctor if you think he or she is not going to respond positively to such news, though, of course, you can if you are unsure about the effectiveness of the treatment and would like to get your doctor's opinion.

Hospice

Alzheimer's is not like cancer, where doctors sometimes tell a patient that they have X number of months left to live, but as someone with Alzheimer's gets into the later stages, there may come a time when a recommendation that hospice care is available will be presented to you. Normally, hospices won't accept patients without a diagnosis that he or she has six or fewer months to live, but if hospice care is available, it might be an option you should consider.

Hospice care is gentler than hospital care, as the staff isn't trying to prolong life, but is just trying to make this last phase in a person's life as comfortable as possible. Many patients with dementia become more agitated in a hospital because of all the noise and activity, while a hospice will be more soothing. Medicare will cover most of the costs, and if you are at your wit's end, putting your loved one in a hospice may be the right solution for you. You can even use hospice care as a respite, as you can always ask for your loved one to return home to you after you've regained your strength.

Because a patient with severe Alzheimer's cannot legally consent to hospice care, this option will be open to you only if you have had the proper forms (healthcare proxy, durable power of attorney, living will) signed while your loved one was still able to do so.

Death

Alzheimer's is the sixth leading cause of death in this country. The cause of death for most people with Alzheimer's is malnutrition, as eventually they can no longer eat. Their brain loses so much function that the person can no longer chew or swallow. However, if a feeding tube is inserted, someone with Alzheimer's can continue to live for quite some time. But in many cases, it is the family, usually the caregiver, who must make the decision regarding life and death. The doctor will offer the option of a feeding tube, and if the decision is not to have this procedure, the patient will probably pass away within a week.

As if it weren't bad enough that a caregiver has to devote years to fighting the ravages of this awful disease in someone they love, Alzheimer's gets in a last blow by handing the decision to end this person's life to the caregiver. Once again, the only way to soften this blow is to talk about this at the very beginning and have the person with the disease proactively decide the terms of their final days. The caregiver may still feel bad when giving the order not to insert a feeding tube, but at least this person will be able to take some consolation in the fact that they are carrying out their loved one's wishes.

Alzheimer's is a disease and, like any medical condition, it's natural to turn to the medical community for help. But there's no cure for Alzheimer's and, in fact, the few options for slowing it down aren't very effective. So, the reality is that you, the caregiver, are mostly on your own. The best piece of advice I can give you with regards to medicine and yourself is to make sure that you do whatever is necessary to maintain your own health. Yes, you have to do everything you can for your loved one, but the real health priority is for you to stay healthy so that you can continue to function effectively as a caregiver.

9

Tips for Caregivers

We've covered the basics of what the medical community can do for your loved one, but there are lots of other ways of assisting someone with dementia. Obviously, each person affected with dementia is different, so not all of the following advice will apply to your situation. But, hopefully, you'll find some tips in this chapter that will be helpful, especially combined with some added advice from me.

THE ROLE OF ENVIRONMENT

As a caregiver, you are in charge of your loved one's environment, and, to some degree, this is the most important aspect of the care you provide. The best way to convince you of this is to talk about one place I visited, the Hebrew Home for the Aged in Riverdale, NY. They call their Alzheimer's unit Memory Care Services, as they believe, and rightly so, that each of their patients still has some reserves of memory, and they look at their job as trying to keep their patients in the best frame of mind possible, rather than to just watch them slowly fade away. They try to maximize the faculties that their residents still possess by providing an assortment of different options and treatments, including yoga, aroma-therapy, pet therapy, art therapy, massage, meditation, breathing exercises, and even laughter. The idea is to try to jiggle their residents' circuit breakers in order to get whatever circuitry is still working in their brains to function.

Before you express your doubts as to whether all this can work, Brookdale Hospital funded a scientific study, complete with control groups, over a period of eighteen months, and the study found that patients with Alzheimer's who received these various treatments became much improved in such areas as sleep patterns and behavior.

Understand, all this therapy is not going to halt the deterioration caused by Alzheimer's. The patients studied were all in early to moderate stages of the disease, and eventually all would succumb to it. But as a caregiver, you know that what makes your day most difficult is when your loved one acts up, especially at night, which interferes with your own sleep. So, knowing that there are ways of controlling this type of behavior, without resorting to drugs, is important.

Part of the reason that those Alzheimer's patients at the facility at Riverdale don't act up has to do with the design. The area in which the Memory Care facilities are housed is fully carpeted, bathed in soft light, and all the doors are locked. This allows the residents to roam freely. The staff at the Hebrew Home believe that much of the agitation in Alzheimer's patients is caused by frustration from being cooped up. But having the freedom to roam the halls and socialize with the other residents relieves their frustration and so keeps them from becoming agitated.

How can what goes on at the Hebrew Home help you? First of all, I believe it tells you that you must adopt a holistic approach. You have to examine your loved one's surroundings and see what you can do to lessen the ways in which the environment might frustrate him or her. You also have to provide the means for your loved one to release the frustrations that are inherent in losing one's mental faculties. You have to provide stimulation in ways that, after some experimentation, you notice offer solace to your care recipient.

Specifically, you might try burning a scented candle or incense to stimulate his or her sense of smell. You should try to find scents that are pleasing, but try to vary the scents so that they provide mental stimulation, rather than always using the same scent. If you don't have a dog or cat, you might see if you could borrow one for a time to determine if your loved one gains some benefit from the company of a companion animal. If so, you might consider getting a pet of your own. (If you know any other families caring for someone with Alzheimer's, perhaps you could all share a pet.)

Since your home won't have the same amount of space as a facility, make sure that your loved one gets the chance to exercise, which for the most part will mean going for long walks. I'm sure that you'll be able to tell by the reaction of your care recipient that going out for a walk is a time that he or she craves. If you don't have the time or strength to accompany your loved one, hire a student to come after school and take your loved one for a daily stroll, even if it's only around the block a few times. By the way, I was told of a facility that had a street scene painted on the walls so that when patients would walk around they would feel that they were outside. You might also try taking you loved one to a yoga class for seniors.

Art therapy can mean nothing more than sitting your loved one down in front of a coloring book or giving them some PlayDoh to form into simple shapes. It was actually the artist Matisse who discovered that people with dementia retain their ability to recognize shapes, so your care recipient may appreciate any form of "art" that you give them an opportunity to partake in.

The Hebrew Home actually adopts the Montessori method of childhood education, which takes into account each student's level of ability when setting curriculum. While you shouldn't infantilize your care recipient, you should keep track of how much he or she is capable of doing and offer tasks that will match their ability and even challenge them.

It seems that the more effort you put into finding ways of keeping your loved one active in a variety of different ways—smelling, hearing, touching, moving—the more you'll be rewarded by a lessening of agitated behavior. Of course, as the disease progresses, your care recipient will lose certain abilities. So, while you want to offer challenges to keep your loved one's mind occupied, you have to maintain a certain vigilance to make sure that an activity that once brought pleasure isn't now causing frustration.

You should definitely take cues from your loved one's past. If your grandfather enjoyed watching baseball games, take him out to watch the Little League games in your neighborhood. He'll enjoy getting out and being in the fresh air as much as watching the game, but that's the point. If he played the piano, he might still enjoy doing so, even if the tunes are simple ones. If you play, too, then maybe you could do duets. Hey, even playing "Chopsticks" might be fun.

If your grandmother would enjoy helping out by doing the dishes, let her, even if you have a dishwasher. It will occupy her and playing around with hot water stimulates the senses. If you're worried about her breaking plates, or breaking a glass and cutting herself, buy some plasticware. However, don't let her clean any sharp knives. If it turns out that after she's done the dishes they still aren't clean, stick them in the dishwasher. If she starts washing the dishes but gives up half way through, forget about it. The point is if your loved one will take pleasure in an activity, and can't be hurt, then let her, much as children are allowed to play with pots and pans. The more flexible you are, the easier it will be on everybody.

Some activities may spring to the mind of your loved one on her own, such as heading to the sink to do the dishes after a meal. But others may need to be planned. Your father might actually enjoy a simple task like sweeping the kitchen, but would never think of it himself. So, see what happens if you hand him a broom and say, "Dad, care to sweep the floor?" If he goes for it, great. If not, try to substitute some other activity.

The experts will tell you to plan out your entire day. It's true that following a routine may be comforting to your loved one, and it could also make things easier for you. But at the same time, if you do the exact same things every day at the same exact time, that might drive both of you crazy. You need to test the limits of your care recipient, because any challenges that he or she has to face will keep them from being too bored. How would you know if your mom would like to play solitaire unless you offer her the opportunity, even if she never played when her brain was healthy.

Another point the experts make is that an activity might be pleasurable for your loved one even if it doesn't seem to be. Let's say your father can no longer read—that doesn't mean he might not enjoy looking at a newspaper. You might not be able to tell why he's enjoying it, but you will be able to tell by the look on his face that it is a positive experience, and if that's so, then make sure to give him the paper every day.

Scientists have been able to discover that people who are in a coma may, in fact, be more aware than it seems. Researchers have been able to communicate with some of them, even though the only thing they can do involves brain waves. While there's no doubt that Alzheimer's will have damaged many of the neural pathways in your loved one's brain, there may still be some that are fully functioning, though your loved one may have no way of communicating that to you. So, learn to read body language, and if it seems like a certain activity brings pleasure or is calming to your loved one, even if you can't understand why that might be, then just go along with it.

If your loved one had a career, keep that in mind when thinking of activities he or she might appreciate. Perhaps there might be some simple activities that would relate to what he or she used to do that would occupy their mind. A math teacher might take comfort in looking at a math textbook or playing with a calculator, if only because somehow it seems so familiar. A doctor or nurse might take pleasure listening to his or her own heart through a stethoscope. A chef might want to help prepare a simple meal. It won't work for every possible job, but if you can think of a way to make it work, give it a try. The same would apply to hobbies—if your mom always loved to garden, let her have a hand in working in your flowerbeds.

TRY TO MAKE IT FUNCTIONAL

At the Hebrew Home, they have a "store." The residents can earn points and then buy things for themselves when the store opens once or twice a week. Most of the residents are very aware of this store and they are eager to participate because they get a kick out of buying the little items that are available. This type of activity is not dissimilar to the times when children play store. So, when thinking of things to do, try to come up with activities that have a quotient of playfulness about them. You shouldn't treat someone with Alzheimer's like a baby, as you must help them to maintain their dignity as much as possible, but we all find games amusing, so try to make a "game" out of certain activities in order for your loved one to get more pleasure from it.

You don't want to tire out an older person, but many people with Alzheimer's still have a lot of energy, and if you don't find ways for them to use up some of that energy, it's only going to make them more restless. Since activities like playing a simple game are not mandatory, you needn't worry if on some days the person you're caring for doesn't seem up to a lot of stimulation. On the other hand, if they never want to do anything at all, that's usually not good, either. The reason may be that they just don't know how to get started, in which case it's your job to show them what to do. If you can never seem to motivate them, that would be something to report to the doctor.

Learning the Language of Alzheimer's

I gave a talk at the Hebrew Rehabilitation Center, which is associated with Harvard. I had dinner with some of the specialists there, and some were kind enough to write to me with their suggestions of material that should be included in this book. One of them, a "Dr. Ruth" herself, mentioned that an anthropologist whose wife was at their facility coined the phrase "Learning the Language of Alzheimer's," and she noted how apropos it is.

We are used to communicating with words, but those in the later stages of Alzheimer's are almost like babies in that they may not understand what it is we are saying. They are more likely to pick up on our emotions, but only if these emotions are broadly expressed. Subtlety will be lost on them. If you want to express happiness, do it with a big smile, not a little grin. For example, if your father is looking for his mother, who died decades ago, don't try to explain to him that she's not around, but instead try to comfort him with a hug. No matter what you try, getting through is going to prove difficult to achieve. The following are some tips on how to best communicate with someone with Alzheimer's:

1. Pay careful attention to your body language. People with Alzheimer's, especially in the latter stages, have problems understanding words. They may do better with sensing emotions, and one way they do that is by looking at the body language of the person talking to them. So, if you've got a smile on your face, that will set the tone for the "conversation," while a frown may make your loved one start to fret, and that will probably prevent your meaning from getting across. Yes, you'll be doing a lot of smiling, but even fake smiles have a way of lifting spirits a bit, so don't resent them.

2. Make certain that you have your loved one's attention. Look her in the eye. If she's sitting down, get down to her level. Say who you are, as she may not know you right away and such cues can be helpful. Also, use touch to make sure that she is focused on you.

3. Obviously, you have to use simple phrases. If you don't get a reaction, don't raise your voice, as that may only frighten her. Instead, repeat what you want to say. And don't use abbreviations or pronouns, as she may not be able to decipher them. Instead, use names and very specific terms.

4. If you ask a question, try to phrase it so that he can give you a yes or no answer. Try not to offer choices. If it's a hot day and you want him to wear shorts, don't also offer him jeans. If you show him the shorts and he rejects them, then show him jeans.

5. You have to learn to listen with your eyes, for just as your body language will be important to getting your message across, the body language of your loved one will also provide you with many cues.

6. Be patient, because you may have to repeat what you say many times. If time isn't of the essence and you're not getting through, stop trying for the moment and try again later.

7. If the conversation is making your loved one upset, try doing something to distract her. If you can focus her attention on something else, like a snack or even just jangling your set of keys, then she'll likely forget what was making her upset and settle down.

8. If your mother is on medication, pay attention to whether she is more communicative at certain times more than others. If you notice that the medication is helping or hurting at certain times of the day, avoid trying to communicate during those times. There may be other factors that make certain times of the day better, like after a nap, when her energy level is high.

9. Try to end every conversation on a positive note. It may be hard to tell whether your loved one actually got the message or not, as sometimes she may remember things that never actually happened. But if the overall feeling of an activity, like a conversation, was positive, that will have a more lasting effect.

10. When you're talking to her, keep other distractions at a minimum. Definitely turn off the TV or radio; but you may need to pull down the blinds, as well.

11. Since your care recipient is likely to be of an age when hearing loss may have set in, look for signs that perhaps one reason he is not getting your message is simply that he is not hearing it. If he does have some hearing loss, that is also going to frustrate him, possibly triggering agitated behavior. If you suspect hearing loss, talk to your doctor about it.

12. Your loved one may need time to get her thoughts together, so don't try to initiate conversation when you're short of time. On the one hand, you want to let her talk and don't want to interrupt, but it is all right to fill in a word once you have guessed it in order to keep her from getting frustrated and giving up.

13. If your words are not getting through, be aware that other parts of the brain may be working better than the sections that comprehend spoken language. You might not be able to get a specific message across by singing a familiar song to your loved one, but you might be able to calm them down by offering them something familiar if they're lost in a very unfamiliar world.

14. The same is true with art. A person with Alzheimer's may be able to draw, even primitively, and actually pass on messages, at least in terms of letting you know their mood.

While you will slowly learn how best to communicate with your care recipient, keep in mind that others will not. Your father's physical appearance will not be changing, so other family members who haven't seen him in a while may not realize the changes that have taken place. At family gatherings, you'll have to protect him a bit, and teach other family members how to best communicate.

SOCIALIZATION

One type of person who will know how to communicate with your care recipient will be someone else who has Alzheimer's. At a nursing facility, the residents interact with each other all the time, and this helps to keep them from becoming frustrated. So if you know of any other families taking care of someone with Alzheimer's (and you can certainly find them by joining a local support group), try getting your loved one together with one or two other people with Alzheimer's. Hopefully, this type of socialization will be enjoyable and will have a calming affect. If that is what occurs in a facility, why shouldn't it work for you?

BEHAVIORAL ISSUES

While it is possible to teach a child to follow rules, as the child's mind is maturing and learning to make connections, the exact opposite is taking place in the mind of someone with Alzheimer's. If the person in your care

is acting up or not obeying you, enforcing discipline is going to be difficult and perhaps harder and more frustrating on you then anything else.
Again, that word "flexible" comes into play. You have to keep your loved
one safe, so at times you will have to be inflexible, but most of the time it
is better to bend like the blade of grass than stand firm like the oak tree.

One example I've read about is that of someone with Alzheimer's
who insists on sleeping on the floor rather than in their bed. First of all,
you probably can't guess why they want to sleep on the floor, and they
can't tell you. If it appears to be linked to a fear of falling out of bed, you
could potentially place a rail on the side of their bed, but you could go
to the trouble of doing so only to discover that was not the cause, and
then what will you have gained? The most pragmatic solution is to put
their mattress on the floor, so that they'll be comfortable, and let them
sleep there. Tell yourself that at least you won't have to worry about them
falling out of bed.

The bottom line is that since it is easier for you to change your behavior
than to change theirs, it is better to find ways of accommodating their
wishes than having constant struggles. That's not to say that you shouldn't
try to track down the cause of some change in behavior. There is a reason
why your loved one is acting up, and perhaps if you find the cause, you
can instigate a change. For example, it's possible that the medication that
your mother is taking is making her dizzy. A change in medication might
help, which is why you should report such changes in behavior to your
doctor. You should also discuss these issues with other family members
and friends, because even if you can't spot the cause doesn't mean
someone else won't have a helpful suggestion.

By the way, you could try to see if other caregivers have run into a
similar behavior pattern and see if a solution is available by checking
online at various websites that have boards where members exchange
information. Just because one trick worked for one person doesn't mean
that it will work for you, but there are plenty of ideas out there, many of
which you probably wouldn't come up with yourself. For example, one
common tip offered to caregivers whose charge is prone to what's called
"wandering" (leaving the house and taking off on their own), is to place a
black rug or mat in front of the door. Many people with Alzheimer's will
perceive that rug as a hole and so won't approach the door. I don't know
who first discovered that trick, but it's a very useful one and probably not
one you would have thought of on your own. You can also disguise a door

in other ways, such as attaching a poster to it so that it will appear to be an ordinary wall.

It seems losing depth perception is one common side affect of Alzheimer's, so there may be many other ways in which this plays out that you might not realize. For example, if your care recipient refuses to get into the bath, it might be because he or she can't tell how deep it is and is worried about it being too deep. Thus, whenever your loved one acts in a way that doesn't seem to make sense, see if you can discover if there is a "good" reason for their actions, at least from their viewpoint.

Other ways to deal with wandering include repositioning your locks either higher or lower than normal. A person with dementia may not think to look there. You could also install a lock that requires a key to open it from the inside, but this option carries the risk of not being able to get out if there is a fire or other emergency. You would then have to keep a key near to the door, within everyone's reach, including any children you might have in your home with you. There are also plastic covers that you can place over a door handle that are meant to keep children from being able to open the door (you have to squeeze the plastic cover in order to get a grip on the door knob), and this may work. Sometimes simply putting a sign on the door that says "Stop" will keep your loved one from leaving. And, if no solution seems to keep your loved one from leaving from time to time, putting an alarm on all your doors will at least alert you that the door has been opened and your loved one may be heading out. (If your care recipient doesn't sleep well and so keeps you up, you might have a tendency to take a nap during the day. That might give your care recipient the opportunity to wander off, so that's another good reason to have an alarm on the doors—you'll wake up and know that something is amiss.)

It's also possible to put a tracking device on your loved one, a GPS gizmo that will allow you or the police to find them if they got lost. To me, this would only be appropriate for someone who is in the early stages of Alzheimer's, is able to go out on their own, but occasionally loses the ability to get back home. Otherwise, it would seem to me to be a better idea to do everything possible to keep them by your side. On the other hand, putting an ID bracelet on them, or sewing name tags in their clothes, or at the very least making sure there is a piece of paper in their pockets with their name, address, and phone number would be a good idea. You can also register your loved on with the Alzheimer's Association Safe Return program, which will help the police locate them.

By the way, there are some caregivers who worry that if something should happen to them, for example, if they were in a serious car accident, their loved one might be at risk, so they wear bracelets that say they are a caregiver and their loved one is at such and such an address and who to contact in an emergency.

When searching for a wanderer, it's been discovered that they follow certain patterns, such as following fences or power lines. You might also have to play detective, thinking backward in time, so that if they used to work downtown, see if their goal isn't their old place of employment. It also seems that they are more likely to wander off in the direction that the door they used to get out faces, so use that as a clue.

AGITATION

One reason that your loved one might want to wander off is if they feel agitated, which is fairly common among those with Alzheimer's, as they become frustrated with their condition and especially the way they interact with their surroundings. The best way to deal with agitation is to keep it from happening. Keeping to routines and making sure that everything your loved one uses, like glasses or the TV remote, is always in the same place may help. It will also help if you reduce clutter in the spaces he or she use most, so that a sense of normalcy prevails.

Some agitation is caused by delusions. Your care recipient may have problems distinguishing between what is going on in his head and reality. When this happens, don't merely dismiss what he is seeing, but try to offer comfort, because to him it is real. On the other hand, be careful of what he may be watching on TV, because he might not be able to understand that what he is seeing is not real and that may cause him to be anxious.

In an Alzheimer's patient's weakened mind, delusions can be triggered by other physical problems, such as a urinary tract infection or a toothache. The patient may not be able to explain that this other problem exists, and so rather than complain about the discomfort, what is exhibited is delusional behavior. This means when your loved one seems to be suffering from delusions, you have to be very attentive to everything that he or she is doing. Even though your mother can't tell you that she has a toothache, you might notice that she's not eating certain foods, or that perhaps she's staying away from the cup of tea she usually loves because the heat is setting off pain. Or maybe she's holding her cheek. You might have to make an educated guess that she does have a toothache and take her to a dentist. I know, this is quite complicated, but if you can discover the root of a problem like this, the source of the delusions will go away, and both she and you will be better off.

SUNDOWNING

Another common syndrome is what has been labeled "sundowning," which means that many people with Alzheimer's seem to become more agitated at night. If your loved one is a sundowner, you might also notice more instances of Elder Rage after the sun has set.

The big problem with having the person in your care in an agitated state at night is that you can't sleep. Sleeplessness can make your job much worse and is a serious issue. Here are two different approaches to this problem.

One is to find a place that offers care during the night instead of the day. The Hebrew Home at Riverdale initiated such a program. In order to help those taking care of patients with dementia who were suffering because of the lack of sleep, this facility started a program where they pick up seniors who are sundowners and take them to their facility for the night, making sure that there is plenty to do to keep them occupied, which will automatically be the case because there are other sundowners there. (If you want to read more about this program, you can find an article in the *New York Times* at www.nytimes.com/2009/06/14/nyregion/14cover.html.)

Not only does this program allow the caregiver to get a good night's rest, but because their care recipient will have been up all night, he or she is likely to sleep during the day, giving the caregiver time to do other things. If you don't live near a facility that offers something similar, see if other caregivers in your area are struggling with the same problem, and if there are enough of you so that you represent a significant demand, you might be able to convince a facility in your area to start a nighttime program.

The other approach is a combination of medicinal and behavioral therapy. Hopefully, you'll never feel the need to ask your doctor to give your loved one so much strong medication that he or she becomes like a zombie. It also may not be obvious what the proper dose of medication is for the person in your care. Even doctors admit that figuring out what combination of medications will bring about the best results is an art and not a science. Thus, in order to find the right combination, your doctor may have to make a series of adjustments. Rather than get upset with your doctor for this, encourage your doctor to try various approaches. Try to work with your doctor by taking notes and telling your doctor exactly what changes in behavior, both good and bad, any latest combination of drugs has caused. By working together, hopefully you'll find just the right combination that will keep your loved one from being overanxious while still maintaining their alertness.

Some caregivers don't like the idea of medicating their parent or spouse, but you have to remember that this is also for you, so that you can get some rest. However, one serious downside to such medication is that it can leave the patient disoriented. If your mother is taking a sleep aid, either she might not wake up to go to the bathroom and will wet the bed, or else she might be dizzy when she does get up to go to the bathroom and thus fall and hurt herself. That's not to say that you shouldn't use such medication, but that you must be alert to such issues. Even if she normally doesn't need diapers, you might want to use them. And you might want to place a baby monitor in her room so that when she gets up to go to the bathroom, you'll know about it and can assist her.

Also, just as you can do with young children, if you keep a sundowner as active as possible during the day, the likelihood increases that he or she will be sufficiently tired at night to fall asleep. So, if sundowning is a problem with your loved one, keep them busy during the day.

You also need to see whether your loved one's diet has any involvement in changes in sleep habits. Try to limit sugary sweets, especially late in the day, as these might be causing them to be more active at night. Also, don't serve the big meal of the day right before bedtime, but rather offer smaller meals throughout the day.

If not addressed, sundowning can turn into a vicious cycle. Your loved one keeps you up at night so you're both exhausted the next day, and so the day goes by quietly, with maybe both of you taking naps, and then that night the pattern repeats itself. That's why you have to take action of some sort right away, or this pattern of being up at night and quiet during the day will become ingrained and much harder to change. Of course, I would suggest employing behavioral techniques first, like keeping your loved one active, but don't hesitate to bring in your doctor to help with medication if behavioral techniques are not sufficient. Sleep deprivation is considered a form of torture, and it will definitely impact your health if it goes on for too long. On the opposite end of the spectrum are those who won't allow a facility to use any behavioral modification medication on their loved one, fearing that it will be abused. While that danger exists, a reputable facility will only administer it for the right reasons. I know of at least one case where a family didn't allow a facility to medicate their mother—she was often aggressive without the medication—and so for the safety of the staff and the other residents, this woman was asked to leave.

Of course, as your loved one goes through changes, the dosage of drugs may have to change, so this may be a never-ending process. Still, because drugs can be so helpful with behavioral issues, it's worth the effort of working with your doctor to maintain the best possible dosage, as in the end you, the caregiver, will benefit.

Let me reiterate that it's very important to report to your doctor any other medications and supplements that you give your care recipient. You may think giving aspirin or any over-the-counter medication has no bearing on your care recipient's condition, and normally it wouldn't. But every medication has an impact on other medications in a person's system, and if the effect is, say, to multiply the effect of one drug, you could make a perfectly safe drug dangerous. So never administer medications, even over-the-counter ones, without checking with your doctor. And if your loved one has more than one doctor, be very diligent about letting each doctor know which medications the other has prescribed.

The important thing is to understand that other caregivers have managed to find a solution to this problem, so you too must do whatever it takes to find an answer that works for you. If you get the idea in your head that you're stuck in this situation, you will be, and that would be terrible. The only solution at that point, for the sake of your health and sanity, would be to send your loved one off to a facility, and if that's something you'd like to put off as long as possible, make sure to take care of this issue as soon as it arises.

Elder Rage

Sometimes, simple agitation grows in intensity, which has been dubbed Elder Rage. For the most part, Elder Rage is verbal—as in a person may scream or use profanity—but sometimes it can become physical, as well. If you're caring for someone who is bigger than you are, this could be dangerous. The rage is an outgrowth of the agitation they may be feeling, but it is exhibited in a much stronger form. The person you're caring for may get very upset with you or with something else, or maybe even seemingly at nothing at all, as delusions can also trigger Elder Rage. Or the cause might be so slight that the reaction far outweighs the source of irritation.

In part, someone who exhibits Elder Rage does so because of a loss of inhibition. When you become upset, you try to control your emotions, especially in certain surroundings. But someone with dementia doesn't have those brakes. A person with Alzheimer's will express all their emotions without any filters. Since we're not used to that behavior, at least in adults—certainly babies and toddlers don't hold back—it appears to us to be an extreme type of behavior. But if you look at the situation in its proper perspective, that of delusional thinking, it will be easier for you to accept these emotional outbursts.

I read a story about a caregiver who kept trying to convince her father's doctor that he was exhibiting Elder Rage, but every time he was examined by the doctor, he was as sweet as he could be, so she wasn't able to convince the doctor that he needed to be placed on medication. She had to look around until she could find a psychiatrist who would put her father someplace where he would be under observation for a long enough period of time that her father exhibited the rage she'd been complaining about. After the proper dose of medication was determined, she also used tough love to keep him in line, not giving him dessert, which he loved, when he acted up, and rewarding him with an extra dessert when he showed good behavior.

I give you this story to show you that it might not be that easy to get the help you need, which is why you have to be persistent. Again, I said the help *you* need. You're kind enough to be shouldering this responsibility, but that doesn't mean you need to be tortured on top of everything else.

There are two other factors about your care recipient's behavior to keep in mind. First, if you have any outside help that comes into your home to assist with caring for your loved one, you might lose a good person if your loved one regularly becomes uncontrollable. You might have no choice but to put up with such behavior, but that's not true of someone you hire. And, if the time comes that you can't handle your loved one anymore, be aware that not every facility will accept someone who exhibits Elder Rage, which might mean the facility you would really like to use will have to be crossed off the list. Doing your best to get this Elder Rage under control could be important if the moment arrives that you need to put your loved one in someone else's care, and you want that to be at the best possible facility.

However, if your loved one is continually showing signs of Elder Rage and you can't seem to control it, at the very least you have to make sure that there is nothing within reach that could be used to harm anyone. You may not have to get a metal detector for your house, but you will have to be vigilant about keeping any sharp instruments out of reach.

If your care recipient does become violent from time to time, and if you are not strong enough to handle the situation, you need to find someone you can call in an emergency to help you. You can call the police, but that might lead to your care recipient being arrested, which is only going to further complicate your life. So, see if you can develop a plan to keep yourself safe when you're faced by Elder Rage that won't involve the police. On the other hand, if you're in a situation where you're in danger and there's no one else to come to your aid, by all means do call the police. Eventually, you may be able to sort the problem out and at least you'll be safe in the interim.

DON'T BE OVERPROTECTIVE

Some cases of Elder Rage are perhaps justified, at least to some extent. If you, as a caregiver, are overprotective, treating the person you're caring for like a baby, and that person retains some capabilities, you're setting yourself up for a negative reaction. Certainly, there are activities that must be curtailed. It seems many caregivers have to struggle to take away car keys, for example. Even the slightest chance that your loved one might cause a car accident is reason enough to enforce a no-driving rule, and, yes, that will cause frustration and anger for a time. But if the two of you have lots of little fights over matters of control, then maybe you're the one who is going to have to compromise. Your loved one is an adult, after all, not a child, and so has many years of being independent. Of course, that's likely no longer fully possible, but you can understand that this situation is frustrating.

If your mother wants to dress herself, don't worry if she tends to put on older or less fashionable outfits. If she likes a certain yellow blouse and it's becoming frayed, see if you can't find one that is almost like it and buy it for her, rather than fight with her over what she's wearing. Yes, she's not being entirely rational, but just because you're technically right doesn't mean that the two of you need to argue over what she wears every day. In the long run, these minor battles will eat away at your resources, and you need to manage them carefully.

At some point, you might begin to feel that you're always giving in, and out of frustration you dig your heels in and try to assert as much authority as possible. The problem is that you're not dealing with someone who is fully rational. And, if your loved one is bored, fighting may be a way of relieving that boredom, so it's just not a struggle that you can win.

Every book and website aimed at caregivers tells you that, rather than struggle with your care recipient, you have to keep a smile on your face, because the person you're caring for will pick up on your feelings. If you won't argue with them, they'll soon stop trying to start an argument. That's certainly good advice, but at times it's going to be hard to follow. It won't necessarily even be the fault of the person you're caring for. You could be exhibiting sadness for some other reason than being a care-giver, or perhaps the loneliness of your situation could have you in the dumps.

What do I do when I'm feeling a bit sad? I've got a drawer where I keep old letters and other communications that bring a smile to my face when I reread them. If I'm feeling down, I open up that drawer and spend a few minutes reading the missives I've put aside for just that purpose. I suppose if I was more of a techie, I'd save e-mails in a folder in my Outlook that would accomplish the same thing.

You could also tear out articles you read that bring a smile to your face. Or make a copy of a favorite passage from a book and keep it with you. Uplifting music can also help. Make a CD or playlist on your iPod of music that lifts your spirits. Maybe you have some cute footage of your grandchildren that brings a smile to your face. If putting together one DVD of the best of these is beyond your ability, or beyond the capability of your equipment, ask your son or daughter to do it. It's really not all that complicated if you know how. You could even ask your grandchildren to make silly recordings for you.

You'll know best what type of material can lift your spirits, but this is a job you must do before you're feeling low. You want to be prepared to face those bad days with something that will make you feel better as quickly as possible. Once you get started, it will be easier to add to your collection, but you have to make that initial first step.

You should also make a list of friends or relatives who know how to lift your spirits and keep that list handy so that you can make a quick phone call. Sometimes, a five-minute call will really make a difference and allow you to get through the rest of the day. (On the other hand, if there's someone who brings you down and their number comes up on caller ID, let the call go to your answering machine.)

By the way, you might think of changing the message on your machine to add that sometimes you won't pick up because you're too busy taking care of your loved one. That way, if you don't pick up when a caller expects you to be home, that person will be less likely to worry and you'll feel less guilty about letting your machine pick up your calls.

You also need to pay attention to your environment. If you're lacking light, then either move outside, or open all the blinds, or turn on a bunch of lamps. Lamps are available that specifically mimic daylight, so sitting under one of them might be helpful, especially in winter when it's harder to get outside. The air inside your house can also bring you down, so open the windows and let in some fresh air. If the air is too dry in winter because of the heating system, use a vaporizer. Both you and your care recipient will benefit.

It might also be helpful to look at your loved one differently, especially if he or she is the source of you being in the doldrums. Maybe just going over and giving them a hug would help lift both your spirits. Or, if there is something that you know gives them joy, do that activity together. Maybe just make silly faces at them, which will take out some of your aggression without actually fighting with your distressed loved one.

ELDER-PROOFING YOUR HOUSE

I've mentioned some tips with regard to maintaining a house environment for someone with Alzheimer's, but you should really look at every aspect of your home to make sure that there is nothing dangerous in it and that it is as easy as possible for your care recipient to manage. For example, your mother might forget where things are, but she still might be able to read, so if you put labels on things, this could be helpful to her. I'm not just talking about drawers, as in "Socks," but even items that are quite visible, like the toilet. She might not recognize the toilet for what it is, but if she is able to read a sign that says "Toilet," a light will go on in her brain and she'll use it.

If you keep the temperature in your hot water high, lower it so that your care recipient won't accidentally be scalded. Take a careful look around your kitchen and make sure that nothing dangerous is in reach. This can be more difficult than with small children because, while they're not tall enough to reach many things, your care recipient is. You might want to add an automatic shut-off switch to your stove, which may be annoying to you at times, but could prevent a serious accident.

Lighting is also important, both inside and outside of your house. Older people are always prone to falls, but that's especially true of those with Alzheimer's, so the better lit your surroundings are, the less likely an accidental fall. That is also true of any type of clutter. If you have any children around the house, make sure they understand how important it is not to leave their belongings lying around. Any inherently unstable furnishings, like scatter rugs, should also be removed.

REPETITIVE BEHAVIOR

One common aspect of dementia is that your loved one may repeat certain questions or actions over and over. To some extent, this is to be expected with short-term memory loss. You may have answered this particular question one minute ago, but as far as you loved one is concerned, she never got the answer and so she asks it again.

There are two main ways of handling this type of situation. One is to write the answer down, like what time dinner will be served, and leave it someplace apparent. You might even place a chalkboard in a prominent place where you can write down this type of information. If that doesn't work, you'll have to try to distract your loved one's attention to another subject. If the question is about mealtime, a little snack might work, as she won't feel as hungry. Or, introduce an activity that will be distracting.

The one thing you shouldn't do is tell your dad that he just asked that question. He won't remember, and it will only make him more anxious. If you don't have time to do something distracting, it's probably simpler just to answer the question again and again over the period of time that question remains in play.

If, instead of asking a question, your loved one is doing something else over and over—picking at a shirt and obviously demonstrating anxiety—try to see if you can discover the source. If, for instance, your dad needs to go to the bathroom, helping him do so might end that repetitive behavior.

EXERCISE

Another type of repetitive behavior is pacing. On the one hand, exercise is a way of reducing stress, but too much can cause physical problems on joints, not to mention on your nerves. Taking your loved one out for a walk, even one of over an hour, might reduce the pacing, and it would be good for your health, too. Keep in mind that constant pacing can be an intermediary step to wandering, so make sure that you take the necessary precautions that I've already mentioned if it appears that pacing might indicate an urge to wander.

It's been shown that walking can actually slow down the advance of Alzheimer's, so by taking your loved one for a walk every day, you might actually be helping to keep both of you healthier.

While an electric treadmill might be too dangerous for your loved one, some are available that are strictly mechanical, meaning it's the person's feet that move the tread, not a motor, and so if the person stops walking or falls, there are no moving parts to injure anyone. Placed in front of a TV, this might be a way for your loved one to "pace" without actually moving through your house.

If, however, your loved one seems unwilling to move about—and not getting enough exercise can certainly have an adverse affect on his or her health— see if you can discover the cause of the inactivity. There are a few reasons that might not be readily apparent—a loss of balance, poor vision, pain in one leg—that might be cured by the use of a cane. You might try offering a cane and seeing if that helps to get your loved one to move around more.

You may think of exercise as being important for your care recipient, but there may be a side benefit for you—better sleep. Though you don't want to tire her out completely, if you make sure that she gets enough physical exercise every day, it will likely help her to sleep better. If the weather doesn't permit going outdoors, some malls have early morning group walks, or else you can look for a day-care facility for seniors where she will have a chance to move around.

EATING

Depending at what stage of Alzheimer's your loved one is in, you may run into different sets of problems regarding eating habits. Some people with dementia regularly forget to eat, and they may lose too much weight, while others will forget they just ate and so eat again and be liable to an unhealthy weight gain. Even with a loved one in the early stages of Alzheimer's, you have to keep careful watch.

If your loved one is capable of feeding himself or herself, allow them to do so, even if the process is a bit messy. If it helps, cut food into small pieces and allow them to eat with their fingers. For drinking, use straws or a child's sippy cup. Older people, even those who do not have Alzheimer's, often don't drink enough and risk becoming dehydrated, which may cause constipation and other health problems, so be certain that your care recipient is getting enough liquids during the course of the day. If the weather is warm, or if your home is dry in winter because of the heat, it's important to increase their liquid intake.

As the disease progresses, you may find that you're going to have to encourage them to perform such necessary tasks as chewing (by helping them to move their mouths up and down) and swallowing (by gently caressing their throat), so while you may not love the messiness of one stage, you need to appreciate it for what it still allows your loved one to do on their own.

It's likely you're going to have to prepare special meals for your loved one; for example, if chewing is difficult because of dentures, he or she will need softer foods. But just because your mom is getting a separate meal doesn't mean that she should eat alone. Eating a meal is usually something we do together, so if she can't sit down at the dinner table with the rest of your family, try to have at least one person sit with her while she's eating.

People with Alzheimer's regress in so many ways, and one way, worth seriously watching, is in their eating habits. They seem to prefer salty foods, like chips or nuts, and sugary foods, like ice cream. If they have health problems like high blood pressure, for which salt intake must be regulated, or diabetes, which means their sugar intake must be strictly limited, this can be a problem, especially as they may make quite an effort to get at such forbidden foods. If that's the case, you won't be able to keep these foods in the house. On the other hand, if your husband never liked leftovers, that problem will disappear as he won't remember what he's eaten recently, and you can probably make dishes that you enjoyed and he never did, as he won't remember that he doesn't like that particular dish.

If your loved one always asks for the same favorite dish, as long as it supplies the proper nutrition and is not too difficult for you to prepare, don't worry about the sameness. If having the same dish encourages your loved one to eat, and if he or she doesn't remember that this dish was served the last six nights in a row, by all means, go ahead and humor them. On certain matters, you have to put yourself in your loved one's shoes and not worry about what makes sense to you.

HOLIDAYS

Food and holidays go together, but holidays can be problematic to someone with Alzheimer's for several different reasons. The first has to do with holidays triggering memories of the past, which can be painful, given their current circumstances. Holidays also can mean crowds, which can be disorienting. Try to limit your loved one's time in crowded situations, and if she has to be present, make sure there is someplace you could take her to give her a breather, like a spare bedroom.

While holidays are supposed to be happy times, for some people they can cause the opposite effect—I'm not talking about your loved one, but you. You may feel the burden of being a caregiver more strongly during the holidays because they cause you to remember how your loved one was before this terrible disease struck.

It's important for you to be aware of this potential effect. I've already suggested some ways to help combat the blues, but they can only be effective if you're aware that you are feeling down. So, when the holidays come around, monitor your mood. If you do seem to be more down than usual, then put in the extra effort to actively raise your spirits. If the depression lasts beyond the holiday period, you might want to consult your doctor about it. You can suffer from depression just as much as your care recipient, so don't ignore it.

Personal Hygiene

Personal hygiene often presents problems between the patient and caregiver because of issues of modesty. Your loved one may try to avoid a bath or shower, not because they like being dirty but because they feel very uncomfortable having you involved in keeping them clean. You may not feel any better about it, and your body language may end up being part of the problem. If you're both embarrassed and both react negatively, bath time could turn into a battleground.

If your loved one is worried about falling in the bath, one simple way of alleviating that fear is a pair of bath shoes with non-skid soles. Or, if that's not an option, you can purchase a chair constructed for using in a bath or shower (made of aluminum and plastic with holes in the seat so that the water drains.) Adding a handheld showerhead for your loved one to use while sitting on a chair will make it easier on both of you. You should definitely add bathtub bars for holding on, and it's also possible to convert your bathtub to one that has a door on the side, so there is no danger climbing in and out of the tub. I've already mentioned that many people with Alzheimer's have problems with depth perception, so stepping into a tub can seem quite scary to them.

Some middle ground must be found between cleanliness and safety, as you should never leave someone with dementia alone in a bath or shower. Do everything you can to preserve their sense of modesty, even allowing them to wear a bathing suit if that removes much of their anxiety, but always make sure that you have everything you need in the bathroom, so that you never have to leave your care recipient alone to go get a robe or answer the phone.

Depending on how difficult these experiences are, you may have to allow for longer periods of time in between major washings. Twice a week is probably acceptable for someone who doesn't move around that much and so never works up a sweat. However, if their ability to go to the toilet is limited and they must wear diapers, you will have to clean down there regularly to keep skin irritations from developing.

One method of keeping patients clean in hospitals and other health facilities is the towel bath. The patient is on a large bath towel, and other towels are used to cover the parts of the patient not being cleaned, while a damp cloth and no-rinse soap are used for the actual cleaning. (For more on this subject, read the book *Bathing Without a Battle*.)

One reason that you need to clean someone with Alzheimer's regularly is the issue of incontinence. Incontinence in people with Alzheimer's is often just a matter of forgetting to go, so gentle reminders throughout the day can be helpful. But you won't be there to remind your loved one at night, and the easiest solution is to just start using adult diapers as soon as the problem arises. The odds are that your care recipient won't think twice about it, even though you may hesitate, so rather than delay using them, start right away. You may want to double up on them at night and also place a washable pad on top of the sheets.

For men, make sure that the penis is pointing downward because that's where the absorbent material is located. If it's pointed up, there's a greater chance for leakage.

Tip: When traveling, even just around town, keep a spare set of clothes in the car, just in case there's an accident.

DRESSING

Make getting dressed part of your care recipient's daily routine. Even if you don't plan on going out, don't let him lounge around in his pajamas all day. If possible, try to make getting dressed something that takes place at the same time every day so that he expects it and won't fight you. If he wants to select his own outfit, try to keep the options that are visible to a minimum. If he selects the same outfit every day, just buy a few that are identical so you can wash his clothes without causing a fuss. Using clothes that don't require complicated maneuvers, like buttoning, is usually best. Pants with an elasticized waist, like sweatpants, for example, need only to be pulled up. If he can dress himself, put out the clothes in their proper order, undergarments first. If you're supervising, hand them to him one at a time.

Even if having him dress himself takes longer, let him do it. Try not to show frustration if he's having a particularly hard time with a garment. It's important that he feel some measure of independence, and so if he can dress himself, let him.

Sexually Inappropriate Behavior

If you read about two people with Alzheimer's in a facility who don't have any memories of their spouses and who form a romantic relationship, you might think, "Isn't that cute." But when you're taking care of someone in your home and they act in a manner that is inappropriate, especially if there are children around, then "cute" is the last word that will pop into your brain.

When your care recipient takes off clothes in front of others, or masturbates, or makes remarks about wanting to perform some sexual act, perhaps even in an aggressive manner, that is going to be embarrassing, to say the least. Of course, it's the disease that is at work here, but that doesn't make it any less disconcerting.

One aspect that you have to consider is that those with severe dementia who can't verbalize what they are feeling will exhibit those feelings by acting out. So, if your mother can't tell you that she's hot, she may show you by disrobing. Since she may also have lost her sense of cultural norms, it won't occur to her that being naked in front of other people is not part of our social fabric. The same may apply to a male who exposes himself and masturbates. He no longer has the ability to understand that this is behavior that is not acceptable in public.

Your first line of attack is to let your loved one know, in gentle terms, that this behavior is not proper. Even if this is embarrassing to you, use direct language, because someone with Alzheimer's is much less likely to understand euphemisms. So don't say "Stop touching yourself down there," but instead say "Stop masturbating" or "Leave your penis alone." If one way of saying it doesn't work, try another. But keep in mind that if one phrase works one time, that doesn't mean it will work the next, so always be prepared to give these suggestions using a variety of different wordings.

As with any behavior that you want your loved one to stop, redirecting their attention is certainly the next approach to use. If you can divert your loved one's attention toward something else, there's a good chance that he or she will forget the stimulus that initially caused them to become aroused. If it happens often enough in public, outside of your home, you may want to carry around a loose robe that you can quickly use to conceal him or her. It may also be helpful to dress your loved one in trousers without a fly, like sweat pants, which will make it more difficult to expose genitalia, particularly in the case of men.

You might also consider keeping a diary of this behavior. Take note of triggers. Maybe seeing a certain person triggers inappropriate sexual behavior, in which case avoiding that person, at least in public, may be helpful. The stimulus could even be an actor or actress who appears on a certain TV show. People without dementia can develop crushes on celebrities, so why not someone with dementia? If that's the case, you want to make sure to avoid that program. Also, if you notice that this behavior takes place after a particular medication takes effect, note that too. (Certain antidepressants can, as a side effect, cause a heightened desire for sex.) If your loved one drinks alcohol, which loosens everyone's inhibitions to some extent, determine whether that might be a trigger. In any case, if you take careful notes, you can then inform your doctor and obtain advice about the problem.

If this type of behavior is accompanied by violent behavior, then that changes everything. This is more likely to occur if such behavior has been exhibited at times prior to dementia setting in. Maybe this violent behavior was tempered before dementia, or only brought on by alcohol use, which can be halted, but now it becomes more pronounced because the patient with dementia has lost the control over their temper that they once could maintain. In such cases, you will have to let your doctor know. It may be caused by medications, in which case an adjustment may help; it could also be tempered by medication, which your doctor can prescribe. If the violence puts you at risk, immediately call another relative or the police. If the person you're caring for is prone to violent behavior, always make sure that nothing lethal is within their reach, and make sure that you don't allow your care recipient to get between you and a door to escape, especially if you are female and your loved one is bigger and can overpower you.

Of course, as we all should know, age does not remove sexual desire or the need for sexual release. If your loved one feels the need to masturbate, he or she should be given the privacy in which to do so. It is not uncommon in facilities that two people with dementia will develop a sexual relationship. It is difficult for caregivers in these facilities to be able to judge whether any sexual activity is consensual on both sides, so not every facility will offer those in its care the privacy to engage in sexual activity with another patient. (The potential reaction of the families undoubtedly also plays a role.)

Some male patients exhibit sexual aggression toward any female with whom they come into contact, which means that you cannot have a female come in to give you assistance. There are definitely men who work as home attendants, but to be honest, this is usually a job performed by women, so you may have to do some research to find a male, and the cost may end up being higher as well.

Whatever you do, don't try to hide this behavior from family and friends. First of all, "hiding" may entail cutting yourself off from them, and if you're having to deal with such difficulties, you need more help—physical as well as moral support—not less. So be open about it, explain what has been happening, prepare visitors so that they won't be surprised, and then make the best of it. I'm not saying that this will be easy, but the "easy" way out, cutting you and your loved one off from contact with other people will, in the long run, be much more difficult on you.

VIOLENT BEHAVIOR

While sexual behavior can be very aggressive in nature, there is a tendency toward violence among those with dementia that may have a variety of triggers, not just sexual tension. Research has shown that different types of dementia seem to lead to different types of violent behavior. Those patients who have more damage to the frontal cortex, such as people with Huntington's disease, lose their sense of inhibition, and so when faced with something tempting, like someone of the opposite sex, they may act impulsively, and in ways which are not acceptable. Those with Alzheimer's tend to misinterpret the meaning of what is going on around them, and so they feel paranoid, as well as frustrated by their inability to communicate, and they may react with violence toward actions they interpret as presenting some danger, though that's not actually the case. Those with Alzheimer's who act aggressively are said to be nonimpulsive—they are reacting to something going on around them, which they misinterpret or else overreact to because of their feelings of frustration. This is different from the impulsive acts of those with other types of dementia, who are more likely to be kleptomaniacs, for example, taking whatever they see and want. Those with Alzheimer's tend to be more violent, acting out, as opposed to merely stealing, and the more paranoia they feel, the more they tend to act aggressively.

Your doctor can prescribe the proper medication to help your loved one control his or her aggression, which is why you have to report this behavior to your doctor so that you can get this help. Of course, if your loved one is residing in a facility, you have to be concerned that he or she may be the victim of aggression as well as commit acts of aggression. Studies have shown that violence is occurring with greater frequency in many facilities because the tendency toward violence increases in Alzheimer's patients as they progress toward the latter stages of the disease, and most facilities have a much greater proportion of people in advanced stages rather than early stages.

If your loved one is in a facility, you have a duty to examine them for any signs that show they'd been attacked, like bruises. Some residents in care facilities have been seriously hurt. If you notice any signs of abuse, don't hesitate to immediately bring them to the attention of the staff.

As Time Goes By

As time passes, despite any drugs that your loved one may be on, he or she is going to slip into the next stage of Alzheimer's. The changes you notice may be subtle, but after a while they'll be sufficiently noticeable and there won't be any mistaking what has taken place. This might make you sad, and that's understandable, but you can't dwell on this deterioration. If you let yourself sink into the doldrums each time a new stage or partial stage is reached, you will soon be unable to pull yourself out of the blues. Instead, you have to accept what has happened and move on, learning to adapt to the new conditions of your life together and appreciating the capabilities that your loved one has left. As one person said, you have to learn to live with the new normal, as this is part of the process and will happen again and again.

Easier said than done, you say, and that's understandable. But you can do it. Instead of letting your emotions take over, you have to think like a general or a CEO and map out the new strategies you will need to cope with these changes. The more you look at it from a practical point of view, the more you see these new challenges as hurdles to conquer and the less sad they will make you feel.

However, I want to return to something I said in Chapter 2 concerning feelings. If you try to bury some feelings, you may end up burying all your feelings. If this happens, you may not feel as sad as you might otherwise, but that means you also won't feel as happy. You'll slowly deaden all your feelings, and that is not good. So, while you need to channel your feelings of sadness so they don't become overwhelming, you also need to give in to them from time to time. It's okay to go into a corner and cry for ten minutes. It's actually more than okay, it's good for you to let the sadness out. But there's a difference between relieving yourself of some of the weight of your feelings in a physical form, such as crying, and letting them overwhelm you psychologically. You have to learn to manage your feelings so that you let off some of the pressure from time to time, and then channel your emotions into something more active. It's a balancing act, and it may take you some time to learn how to do it, and occasionally the adjustments will be harder to take than at other times. If the burden becomes too difficult, if you feel as if you're going to break apart, that's when you'll have to start thinking about putting your loved one into a facility. But adjusting to the wall that will slowly be encircling your loved one is not easy for anyone, so don't feel badly or guilty if these rough patches get to you, because they get to everyone in your situation.

10

Where You Can Get Help

As we've seen in the previous chapter, there are plenty of medical options for your loved one with dementia, but this book has been written with caregivers in mind, so in this chapter, I will be covering where you can get help.

I understand that your main concern is for the person in your care, and you should be congratulated for that. But to carry out such duties, you have to be in good physical and mental condition. Obviously, if you're laid up in bed, you can't take care of anybody else, but your mental state is also very important. Someone who is depressed, for example, can barely function, and in this state it's especially difficult to take care of both yourself and someone else who is basically helpless. So, rather than making up excuses as to why you can't get help, I want you to promise yourself that you're going to make every effort to get the assistance you need.

At this point, I could give you all the statistics that show how many caregivers are affected by this or that physical or mental problem. However, I'm not going to do that. I don't dispute the statistics, and they're very useful when you're looking at a situation from afar, like someone in government who is planning a budget for health care. But from your perspective, the health of other caregivers is absolutely irrelevant to your own. All that matters is that you maintain your health to the best of your ability. So, while one of your priorities is quite naturally the health of your care recipient, your number one priority is to maintain your own health.

You Are Not Alone

There are tens of millions of caregivers across the country. Not everyone is caring for someone with Alzheimer's, but a lot of people are, and all caregivers share many of the same burdens. Because there are so many caregivers, there are lots of agencies out there to help you. For example, there's the National Family Caregiver Support Program (NFCSP), which is a federal organization funded under the Older Americans Act. Through this program, you can obtain information about the services that are available to you and how to obtain those services, caregiver training, help in the creation of support groups, individual counseling and respite care, as well as supplemental services to directly assist you in your caregiving duties.

How do you best find out what services may be available to you? Probably the first place you should contact is your local Area Agency on Aging (AAA). You can look this agency up in your phone directory under aging or social services.

You can also call the National Eldercare Locator at their toll-free number, 800-677-1116, which can help you locate the nearest AAA. You can get the same information at www.eldercare.gov. Among the services that you may be eligible for (depending on your income) are homemaker home health aide services, transportation, home-delivered meals, and other types of aid, such as cleaning, yard work, and home repair, as well as legal assistance. Depending on your level of income, you may qualify for government financial assistance for some or all of these services. (For more about financial planning, see the next chapter; to find a caregiver support group, contact the Alzheimer's Association, your local hospital, or the Well Spouse Association, a nationwide group for people caring for spouses or partners.)

Phone versus Computer

Before I go any further, I want to offer some advice to those of you who are not computer literate. Because all organizations that cater to older adults recognize that many don't use computers, either because they never learned how to use them, don't have access to one, or their vision doesn't allow them to use computers, you can definitely obtain a lot of information on the phone, and you can access additional information sent to you through the mail. So, it's not as if you've been forgotten. But there is so much information available on the Internet that it would be worth putting in a little effort to access what is there. If you can do that before you get on the phone, you'll have a much better idea of what you might need help with, either via the phone or in person, thus saving you a lot of time as well as opening up avenues of inquiry. I'm not saying that the operator you get won't be helpful, but there's no guarantee that you'll be given every possible piece of information. However, if you spend time exploring the possibilities on the Web, you'll be better equipped when you make that phone call.

So, how do you go about getting computer access if you're not a computer whiz? The ideal way would be if you could get together with some relative or friend who is computer savvy. If you need to print anything out and don't have a printer, you would probably have to go to their home. (And if you have a laptop, you'd probably have to have access to a Wi-Fi connection, too.)

If you do know the basics of using a computer but don't have your own computer, most public libraries have computers for patrons to use, and the librarian might even be able to help guide your search. Your town might have a community center that also offers the same service. There are also Internet cafes where you can rent a machine by the hour.

If you have problems with your vision, many of these public computers are equipped to enlarge the type on the screen, which may help you. If you're using a friend's or relative's computer, while all computers can magnify to some extent, more modern computers (for example, those that use the Windows Vista or Windows 7 operating systems) can do so to a greater degree.

Finally, if your caregiver duties keep you housebound for much of the day and you're not connected to the world via the Internet, you might want to give serious consideration to purchasing a computer and learning how to use it. Computers are a window to the world, and not only can you find information to help you with your caregiver duties, you can do almost anything else imaginable. Also, with all the social networking possibilities, being able to get online will help you stay in touch with family and friends. Many senior centers, as well as libraries, offer basic courses in computing. Once you pick up the basics, you'll at least be able to do some simple searches that will make information gathering that much easier.

Let me give you an example of something I read on the Internet at a site called Healthboards, where people ask or answer questions or just vent about health problems. One woman, whose husband had had Alzheimer's for three years, was stuck at home because of a snowstorm and had such cabin fever that she was ready to walk away from her duties as caregiver. She posted a message on the boards; others answered her, and at least she got some human contact from people going through a similar problem, people who could completely sympathize with her. It's that type of additional realistic benefit, not merely looking up news about the latest treatments for Alzheimer's, that can make it worthwhile to become computer literate.

Yes, there is a cost involved, but if the only thing stopping you is that you don't know how to use a computer, that's just not a valid excuse. You *are* capable of learning; after all, even toddlers know how to use computers these days, so don't allow a fear of the unknown to be the only thing keeping you from expanding your world in this fashion.

Caregiver Stress Test

The woman I mentioned who was stuck in the house during a snowstorm was under a certain amount of stress, but every caregiver faces stress. The important question is, how much more stress are you able to take before breaking down? If you're not sure how close to your limit you are, you can take a simple caregiver stress test to help you decide. Below is a list of questions similar to what you'll find at Alz.org and other websites that will help you assess your stress:

Which of the following are seldom true, sometimes true, often true, or usually true?

- I find I can't get enough rest.
- I don't have enough time for myself.
- I don't have time to be with other family members beside the person I care for.
- I feel guilty about my situation.
- I don't get out much anymore.
- I have conflict with the person I care for.
- I have conflicts with other family members.

- I cry everyday.

- I worry about having enough money to make ends meet.

- I don't feel I have enough knowledge or experience to give care as well as I'd like.

- My own health is not good.

If the response to one or more of these questions is "often true" or "usually true," you are approaching your limit, and it's time to start looking into how to obtain help. Actually, I would suggest you take the necessary steps long before you reach your limit. First of all, if you can get help, it may keep you from ever reaching your limit, and that may mean that your loved one can remain in your care. But even if sending your loved one to a facility is unavoidable, getting help sooner rather than later may still delay the date, and you'll feel better in the meantime.

As I've said previously, the other reason to learn as much about potential sources of help as soon as possible is that it will be easier to gather this information and make the right decisions if you're not at your wits' end. For example, if you have to interview part-time caregivers, you'll be better able to judge the character of the people you meet if your nerves aren't shot. If you're dying for a break, you're more likely to choose the first person you see rather than call everyone's references. Or else, if you're cranky, nobody will seem good enough. So, don't wait until the last minute. No one can force you to accept help, but at least if you're fully prepared, you'll be able to arrange for help as soon as you require it.

HELPING YOUR LOVED ONE HELPS YOU

Whether or not you're at the end of your rope, are you 100 percent sure that your loved one is getting everything he or she needs to be comfortable? Here's an example I read on a message board, not an official Alzheimer's website: There are the standard medications that are given to slow down the brain deterioration, but maybe your loved one needs other types of medication. For example, one of the problems Alzheimer's patients have is with delusions. Because they are not seeing reality all the time, which can make them very anxious, which in turn makes caring for them even harder. This is not a problem that a regular physician can deal with; it requires a geriatric psychiatrist, who can prescribe medications that will alleviate this problem. You might have been thinking that since your loved one's mind is deteriorating, the idea of taking him or her to a psychiatrist makes no sense, but as you can see, it might. So, yes, do what you can to help yourself with your own chores, but also make a push to see that your loved one is getting the type of care that will also make your job easier.

Speaking of psychiatry, don't think that you might not benefit from some therapy as well, especially the closer you are to the edge. Let's face it: You don't want to burden family and friends with your feelings, especially as your problems don't approach the severity of your loved one's. But similar to the idea that you needn't go hungry just because there are others in the world without enough food, your loved one's problems, or those of anyone else, don't diminish yours. Everybody is helped by having someone listen to them, and if that someone is a professional counselor, he or she can really be of tremendous assistance. Don't assume that you don't need treatment of your own; instead, make the time to get the help that you require.

I've heard of cases where the psychiatrist or neuropsychiatrist of the care recipient also keeps an eye out for the caregiver. Certainly, caregivers are under so much stress that it wouldn't be surprising for them to benefit from such observations. I don't know how common this is, but if you hear of a mental health practitioner who does show this interest, I would advise you to make him or her your doctor of choice.

Of course, that also goes for your physical health. If you're always going to the doctor for your loved one and never go for yourself, stop. You must go for regular checkups, and if you're worried you might have a physical problem, absolutely, without fail, get it checked out. That you're a caregiver is not an excuse to neglect your own health.

Some caregivers who suspect they might have a serious health problem might avoid a trip to the doctor because they say to themselves, "I just don't have time to be sick." While such an attitude is understandable, it's going to cause you more trouble in the long run. People can live for years with Alzheimer's, so it's not as if you can push aside your health problem for a short time until your caregiving duties end. You don't know how long you'll be needed; it could be a decade or more, so you need to take care of any health problems as soon as you note them. The longer you wait, the more severe they'll become and the more likely it will be that you will have to give up your caregiving duties. If you catch a physical problem early enough, there's a good chance that your doctors can help you. But if you let whatever it is fester, at some point it may be too late to get help, or you'll have to undergo such intensive treatment that you'll be unable to be a caregiver for months.

Another thought that may stop you from seeing a doctor is "What if my doctor tells me that I can no longer...." You fill in the blank. It could be anything from "lift my husband out of bed" to "take care of my husband, so he must go into a facility." It's understandable that such a diagnosis is going to cause you to stay away from your doctor so as not to hear it. But your doctor isn't saying this to be unkind, and he surely fully understands your situation (unless you've kept it from your doctor). Your doctor also knows that if you keep doing what you are doing, your condition is going to get so bad that you won't be able to continue as an effective caregiver. So it makes sense to slam on the brakes as soon as possible before your health gets so bad that you'll be physically unable to continue caregiving.

WHERE TO FIND SUPPORT

There's no doubt that you are going through a lot, and there is no group of people who can offer you more in terms of support than other people going through the exact same thing you are. Luckily for you, some of these people have formed small groups, which you are invited to join.

If you're not sure about this whole concept of support groups, it's not something you have to plunge into doing. The organizations that run these groups know how difficult it can be for some to seek out such help, so they've made it easier by providing progressive steps that can help you. The group(s) near you will probably conduct introductory meetings. You'll probably be able to schedule a personal meeting with a support group leader who can answer your questions. If there are several groups in your area, you'll be able to decide which one you might like to sit in on to see if it is the right match for you. These groups are likely to be divided into caregivers for people in the various stages of Alzheimer's, so if you've only recently started down this road, you'd probably want to be with other caregivers whose loved ones have early-stage Alzheimer's, and later you would probably switch to a different group.

If you go into one of these groups with an open mind, I assure you that you will gain an enormous amount of support in so many different ways. The leader and other people in the group will be an enormous fount of information, both about Alzheimer's, but also about the avenues of assistance that are open to you in your community. They can help you find the best doctors, the best facilities, and maybe even the best pizza delivery!

My friend, the famous research doctor, belongs to two such groups. As a professional researcher, he's found that the information he gets from others in his situation has proved to be extremely useful. But more importantly, going to these meetings gives him the opportunity to express his feelings openly, as he knows that everyone else in the room is in the same shoes he's in.

One of the biggest problems that caregivers face is loneliness, and being part of a group can do so much to alleviate this aspect of what you are going through, not just by going to meetings, but also by making friends who will be available to you via phone and e-mail at other times.

Of course, you have to be willing to be open to them, as well. Most caregivers are naturally generous people, but some people are forced into caregiving and may be loathe to share their life with others. Some even seem attracted to the idea of wallowing in their misery. But that is a very unhealthy way to live, and the more reluctant you are to join such a group, the stronger the indication of your need to join one. The human condition demands that we share our lives, especially if we are suffering in some way. It's not good for you to keep it in. Of course, if you have family members and friends who do listen to you, perhaps you don't need to join a support group, though I remain convinced that it would be advisable just for the information you would gain. Unless your family or friends have already gone through this, or perhaps if they were going through it with you, they won't have the expertise to really help you, no matter how much they care about you.

Many caregivers report that their support group has saved their life. They say it's the only place they can go to cry without feeling ashamed. It may also be the only place where they feel they can safely laugh. They look at the other members of their group as an extended family. And, they draw the energy they need to be able to face their daily lives with the positive feelings that are so vital to being a good caregiver. Such groups provide you with the emotional nourishment that can make all the difference between going forward and giving up.

Another potential benefit of a support group is that the members often hand down various goods that have been useful to them at a certain stage when they're no longer needed. For example, if someone's loved one has gone to a nursing home, they no longer need the bath chair, wheelchair, or bedside toilet, and they will gladly pass these on to other members. Since these items can be quite expensive, this is a worthwhile service these groups can provide.

Even if you're reluctant to join a group, I suggest you at least give it a try. It's not an activity you have to immerse yourself in if you don't want to. You can keep to yourself in the beginning, and, trust me, these groups have seen others like you, so they won't be intrusive. But my guess is that you won't sit by quietly just listening for long, because, after a short time, your desire to ask questions and tell others what you are experiencing will swell, and you'll soon find that being an active member of such a group is an important lifeline.

It's certainly possible that there will be people in any group whom you find irritating, or worse. That's just part of any social fabric. But you can find ways to maintain some distance from these people, and it's certainly not worth missing out on this social activity just to avoid having contact with one or two individuals who might be annoying.

In any case, there are no rules that say you have to attend every meeting, but such groups provide a tremendous resource, and, if you stay away from them altogether, you'll be giving up on a lot of information that would be very helpful to both you and your loved one.

One easy way of finding a support group near you is by calling 1-800-272-3900. This is the number for the Alzheimer's Association, and an operator will tell you how to contact the groups that would be most convenient for you to attend. You can obtain the same information by going online to the association website, www.alz.org. The staff of any doctor taking care of your care recipient can probably also give you guidance about contacting local groups, as could any hospitals in the area.

Phone Support

If you can't get out to be part of a support group, or if you'd like extra support, there are phone support groups that you can join. This program is free, but you'll need to register—you'll get a dial-in number and password. To register, call The Legacy at 1-866-644-4944. The phone lines are open Monday to Friday from 9:00 a.m. to 7:00 p.m. Also, the Alzheimer's Association hotline mentioned above, 1-800-272-3900, is manned 24/7, so even if it's the middle of the night and you're at some crisis point and need to talk to someone, you can give them a call.

AFTER YOUR LOVED ONE IS GONE

Losing a loved one is hard for everyone, but the emotions the surviving caretaker of an Alzheimer's victim might undergo can make it an even more confusing time. While you will certainly feel sad, there's a very good chance that you'll also feel happy to be relieved of the burden of having to be a caregiver. That happiness will, in turn, make you feel guilty. For some caregivers who came to actually hate their spouse once the later stages of Alzheimer's had hit, their emotions may make a complete switch, and they find they can once again love the person they married because all the wonderful memories can flood back in and drown out all the horrible ones.

You might think that, once your loved one is gone, you don't need support any longer, but that's not true, and for several reasons. Within a group, you will be able to express these confusing feelings without feeling guilty, because you'll be surrounded by people who completely understand what you are going through, whether or not their spouse is still alive. And, if the people in the group have become like an extended family, you're not going to want to leave them, as that would make the mourning process doubly hard.

There are other grief groups, but in those most of the people you encounter won't have had a spouse who had Alzheimer's, and so they won't be able to identify with you so well. What sets you apart is that you've already had years of mourning. As your loved one went through each stage of the disease, he or she died a little bit more. Your sense of relief, for your loved one as well as for yourself, will be much higher, and so you might not fit into a standard support group for those who are grieving.

I would certainly advise any widow or widower to keep attending the support meetings of the group to which you belonged, at least for a while. I'm sure that there will come a time when you are going to stop going, as you start your life over and don't want to be reminded of how hard those years of being a caregiver actually were. But in the initial months, continue going, slowly weaning yourself from the company of the other support group members. Sadly, there will be new members to take your place, and you may not want to relive your own sad memories each time they reveal their trials and tribulations. (I actually think that individual support groups should have occasional meetings for alumni, which would focus on the future rather than the past.)

Help is available, but just because it's out there won't help you if you don't make an effort to get the assistance you need. Of course, the ultimate assistance is to pass on the care of your loved one to professionals on a full-time basis, which we'll cover in the next chapter.

11

Facilities

At some point, there will probably come a time when you are no longer able to act as caregiver. This might be because you can no longer physically, psychologically, or emotionally handle the duties, or because your care recipient has deteriorated to a point where only institutional care will do, or a combination of factors. This is a painful decision, which I've already gone over, but once it has been made, you have to move on and figure out how best to integrate yourself with the facility.

You might assume that you will be going to this facility as often as possible. But in cases where your loved one has forgotten about you, your visits may only cause him or her a lot of agitation. In some instances, it is a good idea for the caregiver to take a break from visiting their loved one, just so that he or she can get settled in. What is harder to deal with is when your loved one lets you know that he or she doesn't want to be there and makes a scene when you prepare to leave. If you're an experienced caregiver, you know that while you're together you just have to be as warm and comforting as possible, and then when it's time to go, don't make a fuss that will cause more agitation, but just leave quickly, hoping that, given your loved one's lack of short-term memory, your disappearance won't have a lasting effect.

One thing you must be careful about during your visits is referential conversations. Your loved one may not appear to understand what you are saying, but when dealing with people with Alzheimer's, the word "understand" may have different meanings. Even if it doesn't seem that he or she can grasp words, grasping the significance of what you are saying might still be possible. So, if you need to talk to a nurse or doctor about your loved one, have that conversation outside of their hearing.

Some of these communications with the staff are not going to be pleasant. It is doubtful that any facility can provide all of the personal care that you gave, but, nevertheless, there is going to be a minimum level of care that you want your loved one to receive, and if you feel that he or she isn't getting that, you may become upset. You have to recognize that part of your reaction is going to be fueled by any guilt you may feel for having sent your loved one out of your care. If you've done your homework and placed your loved one in a facility with a good reputation, then to some extent you have to back off. On the other hand, if you see something that is clearly a problem, say, your loved one has developed a bedsore, then you definitely need to speak up. (Examining your loved one for bedsores should definitely be part of your routine, if not at every visit, at least with some regularity.) But since you are not there most of the time, and since your loved one probably can't communicate very well, if at all, you also don't want to create a situation where staff members might take out their negative feelings toward you on your loved one.

This is a situation where it might be good to find an ally so that you can play good cop/bad cop. Let's say you are the one who goes to the facility regularly. You've tried to nicely point out to the staff that something needs to be corrected, but it's not being done. Rather than making a fuss yourself, you could ask another relative or friend to pay your loved one a visit, maybe even at a time when you're not there at all, and let that person take a more adamant stand. Hopefully, they can initiate action, and you won't have spoiled your relations with the staff.

Those relations are important since you can't be there most of the time. You need to have good communication, because if there is some sort of problem, you want to be contacted right away. You want the people there to bend over backward to help your loved one. That means you want to be on friendly terms with the staff. Bringing gifts, and perhaps tips, might help. (You might not be permitted to give individual cash gifts to any one staff member, but many institutions have a fund, for the holiday party, for example, and so you can contribute to that.) But at the very least, you want to be courteous and keep all communication civil. Losing your temper is probably only going to have negative consequences.

If you have any doubts about the quality of care your loved one is getting, I suggest that you do some research on what other options are available. That doesn't mean that you will definitely make a change, but at least you'll be armed with the information you need in case that step is needed. If you discover that there really is no better place—and that decision might be based on a number of factors, including proximity, cost, and the quality of care—then you'll just have to put in more effort and perhaps more money to see what you can do to raise the level of care for your loved one. For example, you might be able to employ some private-duty care for a loved one. I know of a 92-year-old man without a family, whose mind is fine, but who is lonely and loves it when a private-duty massage therapist comes in and puts cream on his skin, which is very dry.

I'm all for fighting battles, but only if you are sure that either you can win the battle or bear the cost of losing it. Even if your loved one is not in your actual care, you still bear the primary responsibility for him or her, so you have to pick and choose your battles.

In a facility that houses people with Alzheimer's, you have to watch out not only for the staff but for other patients too. Given that so many people with Alzheimer's can show signs of rage or violence, you have to make certain that your loved one is getting adequate protection from the other patients. The level of violence in these facilities is rising as they fill up with more and more people with Alzheimer's. Because someone who seems docile may suddenly turn angry, it's very hard for the staff to anticipate one patient striking another, but certainly when you are there, be vigilant, and if you sense that your loved one might be in danger, speak up.

QUALITY OF CARE

Every caregiver whose loved one is now in a nursing home is concerned about the quality of care that they receive. But so is the facility. The rules and regulations they must follow are strict and ever-changing. The detail that goes into the rules about bedsores, for example, is mind-boggling. Care for bedsores is not paid for by government funding, because hospitals are not permitted to let them develop in the first place. This same set of rules may soon apply to nursing homes. When the rules become more stringent, the cost of care goes up. Thus, everyone is caught in a Catch-22 of sorts, because as the elderly population grows, government funds have to be stretched more and more, and, at some point, we're going to reach a breaking point. But families are also financially stretched to the limit by a disease that requires so much care for such a long time.

Studies have shown that nursing homes tend to use drugs to keep their charges calm in ways that may be dangerous. A government study showed that half of these drugs are being administered when they are not appropriate. You have to be vigilant about which drugs your loved one is receiving and when, then checking with your doctor to make sure that the correct drugs are being used. While you might think that this inappropriate use of drugs is being done just to keep the patients calm so that it's easier on the staff, it's been found that some of this misuse is because of financial incentives that pharmaceutical companies are giving to the facilities, in part because Medicare is paying for these drugs. If the administration of a nursing home accepts kickbacks, who knows what else they are doing to increase their profits at the expense of those for whom they are caring.

Thus, you are faced with a conundrum. On the one hand, you understand that the high costs of care mean that nursing homes are going to be very careful when it comes to providing services, but, at the same time, you know that some are willing to make cuts that are dangerous to their residents just to make a profit. All this makes finding the proper attitude to take very difficult. You have to be vigilant, but, at the same time, you can't have the expectation that a nursing home is going to provide the same level of care that you could when you were taking care of someone you love on a one-on-one basis. The difference in the level of care may not be a negative reflection on the home, but it could be. There is not a limitless pool of funds for taking care of people with Alzheimer's, and so you have to expect compromises, but to what extent?

Over the years, there have been many nursing home scandals, and there will continue to be owners of nursing homes who are only looking to turn a quick profit. The way in which many for-profit nursing homes are structured can be so complex that it is nearly impossible to discover who actually owns them. Congress has even addressed this issue with the Nursing Home Transparency Act. So, yes, there are some aspects of this industry that are shady.

However, your job isn't to try to change a system that is far from perfect, but rather to do the best you can to see that your loved one is getting the finest possible care. You may become angry or feel guilty at times, but don't dwell on such emotions. They won't really help matters, and they'll only drain you of much-needed strength. Yes, you must watch over your loved one even when he or she is not under your roof, but when you see things that need to be changed in his or her care, you must use diplomacy to get what is needed, not a sledgehammer. And, if it seems to be impossible to get the right care, rather than wear yourself out, find another facility.

ASSISTED LIVING FACILITY

Assisted Living Facilities (ALF) do not provide the medical supervision of a nursing home. However, Alzheimer's is not necessarily the type of disease that requires that level of medical care, and having a husband and wife move together into an ALF may provide the assistance one spouse needs to take care of the other.

Some ALFs have a locked ward for those with Alzheimer's or dementia, but whether that part of the facility is the best option is something to carefully examine. The ALF may be doing this in order to make it seem like their facility is adequate for those with Alzheimer's in order to keep its residents, and thus maintain the monthly payments they are making, but the care may not be adequate.

The biggest problem with using an ALF when it comes to Alzheimer's is that the disease will continue to worsen, and there may come a time when the ALF is definitely not appropriate. That would mean making new arrangements, so it might be wise to skip all the technicalities and expenses involved in making such an intermediate step. That's not to say the ALFs aren't good for many people, just that they may not be appropriate when Alzheimer's is in the picture.

There are some facilities, the Hebrew Home in Riverdale, for example, that offer a wide variety of living arrangements. A couple could start off in an ALF, and if one partner needs more attention, he or she could be moved to another part of the facility while the other remains close by, in the ALF. Hopefully, as the population ages, more facilities with multiple options will open up. Those that currently operate tend to cost more than most basic ALFs, and so for most people, the financial side of the equation will probably be a deciding factor. In our next and final chapter, we'll go into what you need to do in terms of financial and legal planning.

12

Legal and Financial Issues

You may have heard that 80 percent of the dollars that go to the average person's medical care over a lifetime are spent during the last twenty days of their life. I don't know that this statistic holds up for those with Alzheimer's, particularly if you include institutional care, considering that people with Alzheimer's can live for a long time and their expenses can start adding up right from the beginning. One reason that caregivers give so much of their time is that time is something many have in greater surplus than money. Yes, they love their care recipient and want them to have the best care, but the financial burdens of Alzheimer's can be overwhelming. Help is available, including financial assistance, but such assistance doesn't usually come without a cost.

Before I pass on any information, I have to begin with a caveat. Because the services and financial aid available to you depend on the state in which you live, I can't make blanket statements that apply to everyone. You'll have to check out for yourself which eligibility rules may apply, if penalty periods exist, and about other factors that depend on where you live. On top of the variety of laws, and how complicated they are, they seem to be constantly changing, and, at the time I'm writing this book, the laws governing this aid seem to be more in a state of flux than ever. So, the best advice I can give to you with regard to what aid is available and what laws apply to your situation is to tell you to consult an elder law attorney in your state. (My co-author's wife, Joanne Seminara, is an elder law attorney in New York State, with the noted firm of Grimaldi & Yeung, LLP. I am telling you this so that you know that I've double-checked the information we're giving you, but I also have an obligation to disclose that Pierre has a vested interest in this field. But the bottom line is that the advice to see an elder law attorney has nothing to do with my own or Pierre's self-interest and everything to do with yours! Also, in this chapter, I've stated some generalities, but the complexities of the laws are such that these generalities may not apply to your situation. In addition to what the laws say, there's the separate matter of how they are enforced. So, consulting a lawyer who is well-versed in this area of the law is really the wise move, and it is certainly a move that might save you a lot more money than it costs.)

The main reason you need to consult an attorney is that, when it comes to financial aid for health matters, the financial side is completely intertwined with the legal side. To start with, if someone is not of sound mind, he or she cannot personally sign legal papers, including those having to do with obtaining aid. Also, lawyers are required to make that determination, meaning that if they see someone with Alzheimer's, they have to decide whether or not that person's mind is sound enough to make legal decisions. During the early stages of Alzheimer's, the patient usually retains sufficient mental ability to sign papers such as a power of attorney, health care proxy, living will, the Health Insurance Portability and Accountability Act authorization, disposition of remains authorization, wills, and other documents such as trusts. In fact, they may retain that ability for years, especially if they are taking the proper medication. But for others, especially those who didn't get their diagnosis until the disease had started to advance toward the later stages, as well as those in whom the disease progresses quickly, the window of opportunity to sign important papers can be quite limited.

There are some legal documents that everyone should have. Although a young person might not need a will, assigning someone as an agent in a power of attorney (POA) could be very important, because anyone can have an accident and find themselves in a mental state where they cannot function. So, for example, if someone were in an auto accident and wound up in a coma, how would their rent or mortgage get paid? They could find themselves fully recovered three months later, but homeless. Considering these factors, even you, the caregiver, need to have certain legal documents in place.

There are people who are afraid of giving a POA to anyone, even a close relative, because they are afraid that this POA might be misused behind their back. But what these people probably don't understand is there are different types of POAs. You can sign a limited POA that will not pose any risks to you while you are healthy, but could protect you against some very complicated problems if something were to happen to you.

In this book, we cannot explain all the intricacies of the law, especially as they differ from state to state, but, suffice to say, when someone has been given the diagnosis of Alzheimer's, or even suspects that such a diagnosis might be around the bend, if they don't have a POA, they should get themselves to an attorney as soon as possible. They should also sign a health care proxy, so that if they have any wishes as to treatment, and later they are not in a condition to make decisions, someone else can enforce their wishes. As to all the other services a lawyer can provide, these are something you need to investigate personally.

POAs cost money. In New York State, they cost even more now than they used to because the form was lengthened to offer more protection to the person signing the POA, so that the POA cannot be misused. But all those complications add to the preparation time and thus the cost. If you don't have a POA and are totally incapacitated, it's possible for family members, or some other responsible individual, to go to court to be appointed guardian. But that process costs a lot more money and is also time-consuming. If you could hear the horror stories of people who found themselves in a hospital without a POA—and experiencing the ensuing consequences—believe me when I say to you that you would run to the nearest lawyer. You probably have all sorts of insurance. Well, a POA is in its own way a type of insurance, with a one-time fee, which in the long run makes it quite cheap.

In Chapter 5, I advised caregivers who are not the spouse, such as children, especially those who may live far away, to meet the doctor when they visit, because sometimes even if you have all the proper paperwork, whoever it is you're trying to convince of that won't heed the regulations. (Just because they should doesn't mean they will, and if you're trying to exercise a POA via long distance, it will be all the harder.) The same can be true in other situations, for example, at a bank. So, if possible, going to a parent's bank, while the parent is still capable of exercising coherent decision, and making the acquaintance of an officer might pay off later on. Even lawyers with a power of attorney sometimes run into brick walls, so when a layman has to run the same gauntlet, getting what you want can be quite difficult at times.

Making Decisions Together

Many of the decisions that need to be made when planning for the consequences of Alzheimer's are best made together as a family. (And, it is important to be inclusive. Rather than just meeting with one favorite son or daughter, make sure all the children are involved so that a consensus may be reached, or else the bickering that will ensue later by those who were left out could upset the apple cart.) The advice of adult children may be invaluable, as all the planning that needs to be done is quite complicated, and they may have an easier time understanding the more complex aspects. But they will also want to respect their parent's wishes, so you want to have these discussions early enough that the parent with Alzheimer's is as lucid as possible, in order to take part in the planning. That's why putting off such family discussions is a mistake. Yes, when you first hear the word "Alzheimer's," you're not going to be in the mood to think about where you are going to be one, two, or five years from now. But that's exactly when you do need to face those decisions, particularly if every family member is going to have an opportunity to share in them.

Estate Planning

If your loved one needs to go into a nursing home, the cost is going to be at least $50,000 a year, and in a place like New York City it can easily soar to $12,000 a month, or almost $150,000 a year. Those are huge numbers, especially when you think that someone with Alzheimer's can live for many years, even when they are in the later stages of the disease. About 5 percent of the population has planned for this eventuality by buying long-term-care insurance, so that these costs are at least partially, if not fully, covered. (Some policies are capped, either in terms of a total cost or number of years of coverage, and so other plans must be made for Alzheimer's patients whose needs go above and beyond any possible caps.) And, of course, the very rich pay for this cost out of pocket. But what happens to everyone else, all the families that just can't afford that amount of money?

The government, through Medicare for short-term home stays that require skilled nursing care and Medicaid for longer-term stays, will pick up most of those costs under certain circumstances. Again, because these costs are shared with state governments, how much funding is available and the eligibility for obtaining this funding depends on which state you live in. Each state has rules regarding eligibility, which I cannot cover in this book, but some federal rules apply nationally, and those I am going to go over in brief.

Medicare is health insurance that becomes available when you attain a certain age (currently it's sixty-five, but that may soon change). Medicaid is more like welfare in that "means" testing is required for eligibility. Under the current Medicaid guidelines, an applicant can keep a limited amount of cash and income, and other assets may have to be spent down with the money going to the nursing facility until the threshold is met, at which point Medicaid takes over. So, let's say the patient had $100,000 in a savings account, and Medicaid only allowed $15,000, the other $85,000 would have to be spent on nursing home care before Medicaid picked up the tab.

A logical step would be to give those assets away, to the patient's children for example, before applying for Medicaid. Logical maybe, but the government anticipated that loophole, so there is a "look-back" period of five years, which means that any assets given away in the five years prior to applying for Medicaid will be considered assets you could have used to pay for care. So, let's say that $50,000 worth of assets were given away within that five-year, look-back period, Medicaid wouldn't start paying the nursing home costs until $50,000 of the patient's money had been paid toward it. (This example is a simplified one, as the entire process of calculating penalty periods and what qualifies as an asset and what doesn't is quite complicated. The important thing for you to know is that there are ways around some of these regulations, but it will take a lawyer's expertise to help you out.)

I've said over and over again that as soon as you suspect Alzheimer's, you need to take action, and since it could take five years, given the so-called Medicaid look-back period, before institutional care is needed, if you take immediate action, some of your assets could be protected. For example, did you know that it may also be possible to get paid for the caregiving done while the patient was still at home, so that the transfer of money is not considered a gift? But you can't do this without filling out the proper paperwork, called a Care Agreement.

Why is it so important that you protect those assets, aside from the fact that they form a part of your children's inheritance? You never know why or when you may need those assets you spent a lifetime saving up. Let's say a husband gets Alzheimer's, and then a few years later his wife breaks her hip and needs a full-time attendant at home for several months. She would need that money, but it would have all gone to pay for her husband's nursing home care. Even though there are ways to legally protect those assets, some people don't feel comfortable doing so because it involves giving up some control. However, since there are ways of maintaining control while also protecting your assets, it makes sense to see a lawyer and discover what your options are. Most lawyers will charge an initial consultation fee, and if you agree to let a lawyer fully prepare all the necessary paperwork, the total amount can be considerable. But you must look at these fees not as a cost but rather as a good investment, since a lawyer can save you hundreds of thousands of dollars in the long run. And, while many people distrust lawyers, many of those who enter the field of elder law are quite compassionate and have a history of serving the elderly far beyond their legal practice. So, while a social worker might be able to help you fill in the various forms required to apply for aid, if you're not careful, you could fall into one of the dozens of traps that could cost both you and your heirs a lot of money in the long run, more than any possible legal fees.

By the way, Medicaid will only pay for services at places that are government certified, and that certification will soon become harder to get, limiting the places where patients with Alzheimer's can go for care that is paid for by Medicaid. Exactly how all of this is going to play out is still being argued in Washington and may change by the time you read this book. Again, because these laws are not only complicated, but ever-changing, the wisest move is to see an elder law attorney who keeps on top of such matters.

Most elder law attorneys are also familiar with other options for funding of long-term care in addition to Medicaid. For example, if the patient is a war veteran, there may be benefits available for long-term care. And, if you are employed, there may be tax strategies that you can follow, allowing you to deduct some of the costs of taking care of your loved one. As a caregiver, your plate is already full. Trying to figure out all the options is truly a daunting task. If you're a younger person, such as the child of the person with Alzheimer's, you may possess the computer skills to do significant research, but even then the maze of agencies and rules is going to take a lot of time to sort through, and you still might not understand the entire picture, or you might miss an important aspect of what can be done. And for an older caregiver who is not computer savvy, figuring this all out may well be impossible.

Let me give you one small example of what I'm talking about. Money that the patient has in a retirement account that is in payout status, meaning he or she is over seventy and must start taking out 10 percent every year (per IRS regulations), does not count as an "asset" according to Medicaid. The IRS and Medicaid also use different tables when calculating life expectancy. Plus, state laws differ. There are so many details like this that can not only make your head spin, but can lead to your making decisions that will end up costing you, or your heirs, thousands of dollars. Do you really want to take on trying to learn everything you need to know to make the right decisions?

All this can get even more confusing when there are blended families. He has Alzheimer's, is married to his third wife, and had children with the first two. Who's in charge? Is there a prenup, and what effect might it have? Are the husband's assets blended with the wife's, or are they separate? The possibilities are almost limitless, and figuring out the right course of action takes a combination of expert legal skills and the wisdom of Solomon. In some of these cases, the best solution is to actually file for divorce, not because the spouses no longer love each other but because any other option is financially ruinous.

As our population ages and the Alzheimer's population grows, paying for the care of people who can't take care of themselves, and who will likely live for a very long time, is going to become more and more difficult for our society. How this will all play out is anybody's guess, but for now, there are ways for you to get help, and I suggest taking advantage of them.

Appendix: Internet Resources

The following are some Web sites that I found worthwhile. I'm sure there are many more, but this list offers you a good place to start.

Alzheimer's Association: www.alz.org

Self Help Community Services, Inc.: www.selfhelp.net

Family Caregiver Alliance: www.caregiver.org

Caring.com: www.caring.com

Needy Meds: www.needymeds.org

Health Boards Health Message Boards: www.healthboards.com/boards/alzheimers-disease-dementia

Topix Alzheimer's Forum: www.topix.com/health/alzheimers-disease

HelpGuide.org: helpguide.org/elder/alzheimers_disease_dementias_caring_caregivers.htm

TheAlzheimer'sSpouse.com: www.thealzheimerspouse.com

Mayo Clinic: www.mayoclinic.com/health/alzheimers-disease/DS00161

About.com: alzheimers.about.com/od/workingwithyourdoctor/a/specialists.htm

University of Missouri-Columbia Virtual Health Care Team: www.vhct.org/case2400/index.htm

HealingWell.com: www.healingwell.com/alzheimers

United States Dept. of Veterans Affairs: www.tomah.va.gov/Caregiver_Support.asp

Family Caregiving 101: www.familycaregiving101.org

National Family Caregivers Association: www.nfcacares.org

National Care Planning Council: www.longtermcarelink.net

Index

About the Authors

Dr. Ruth K. Westheimer is one of
America's best-known names in relationship therapy. Widely known for her honest
and humane approach to human sexuality,
Westheimer pioneered frank sex advice on
radio with her program *Sexually Speaking*,
which premiered in 1980 on WYNY in New
York. Since then Westheimer has become
America's favorite sex expert, giving help to
millions through radio, television, news-
papers, magazines, books and her website,
DrRuth.com.

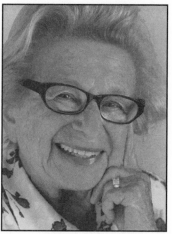

Born in Germany in 1928, Westheimer
was sent to an orphanage in Switzerland
at age 10 to escape the Holocaust. At 17
she emigrated to Israel, where she fought as a scout and sniper for the
Haganah. She was seriously wounded in 1948 during the Israeli War of
Independence.

In 1950, Westheimer moved to France, where she studied psychology
at the Sorbonne. In 1956, she emigrated to the United States. Westheimer
received a master's degree in sociology from the New School for Social
Research and a doctorate of education from Columbia University, and
studied human sexuality under Dr. Helen Singer Kaplan at New York
Hospital-Cornell University Medical Center.

Dr. Westheimer has taught at New York Hospital-Cornell University Medical Center, Lehman College, Brooklyn College, Adelphi University, Columbia University and West Point. She is currently an adjunct professor at New York University and a fellow of Calhoun College at Yale, Butler College at Princeton and the New York Academy of Medicine. Dr. Westheimer has her own private practice in New York and lectures worldwide. She is the author of over 35 books, including *Dr. Ruth's Sex After 50* (Quill Driver Books, 2005).

Pierre A. Lehu has written 20 books, most in conjunction with Dr. Ruth Westheimer, with whom he has worked for more than 30 years. He has also written on a variety of other topics, ranging from fashion to sake.